D0359907

THE 7 DAY SLIM DOWN

THE 7 DAY SLIM DOWN

Drop Twice the Weight in Half the Time with the Vitamin D Diet

ALISA BOWMAN *with the editors of* **Women's Health**

RODALE.

Previously published as an exclusive direct mail edition with the title
The Vitamin D Diet: The Revolutionary Plan That Melts Stubborn Fat Fast in April 2012.

Rodale books may be purchased for business or promotional use or for special sales. For information, please write to:
Special Markets Department, Rodale, Inc., 733 Third Avenue, New York, NY 10017

Printed in the United States of America
Rodale Inc. makes every effort to use acid-free ♾, recycled paper ♻.

Book design by Mike Smith
Photographs by Beth Bischoff

Library of Congress Cataloging-in-Publication Data is on file with the publisher.

978-1-60961-846-9   hardcover

2 4 6 8 10 9 7 5 3 1   hardcover

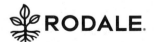

We inspire and enable people to improve their lives and the world around them.
rodalebooks.com

For women everywhere
who are tired of
the annual winter 15

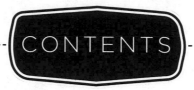

CONTENTS

*I*n 2007, when I became medical director of the integrative medicine program at Northwestern Memorial Hospital, I followed the lifestyle I promoted to my patients. I exercised diligently, ate lots of fruits and vegetables, kept my weight where it should be, and managed stress well.

Vitamin D deficiency was getting buzz, particularly in the holistic health world. During my annual visit to my doctor, I requested a vitamin D test. I'm not sure who was more surprised—my doctor or me—when the test result was 17 ng/mL, significantly deficient, since the normal range is 30 to 100 ng/mL (the ideal is between 40 to 60 ng/mL or more). But really, why was I surprised? I live in Chicago, known as the windy city, not the sunny city, and work indoors all day. But when my D level eventually rose, I noticed a significant increase in my energy, so I am now as vigilant about monitoring my own D level and intake as I was about my old lifestyle.

I began checking the vitamin D levels of my patients, and the vast majority—more than 85 percent—were below 30 ng/mL. I then witnessed dramatic changes in my patients as their vitamin D levels rose into the optimal range. Women who had been diagnosed with fibromyalgia for years suddenly became pain-free; women with depression felt more hopeful; and, overall, women noted greater energy, healthier weight, stronger nails, and thicker hair.

As this book points out, whole foods are the best way to maximize digestion, absorption, and utilization of key nutrients. *The 7-Day Slim Down* provides a core, balanced menu plan, and a flexible approach to exercise.

Vitamin D deficiency and obesity are both epidemic in our country. *The 7-Day Slim Down* provides a plan that can help people feel better, lose weight, and prevent disease. I know I will be sharing the information in this book and recommending the diet to my own patients.

—*Melinda Ring, MD*
Medical director of Northwestern Integrative Medicine at Northwestern Memorial Hospital in Chicago and coauthor of The Natural Menopause Solution

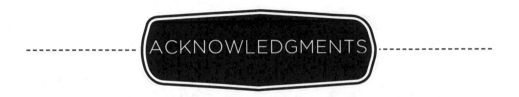

ACKNOWLEDGMENTS

I'm indebted to Bridget Doherty, a former senior editor at *Women's Health* magazine. Several years ago, she called, told me that vitamin D was the next wonder vitamin, and assigned me the story that eventually led to this book.

I'm just as indebted to Ursula Cary, my editor at Rodale, who saw the need for this book long before I did. Ursula is a rare gem, the kind of editor every writer needs. Not only did she help to polish the manuscript, she consistently alerted me to research that I might want to include. She's much more than an editor and a wordsmith. She's also a strategic thinker and trend spotter. I consider myself blessed to have written under her guidance.

To the dozens of women who agreed to test this diet before it went to print: thank you. It was through your feedback that I was able to see which recipes worked and which ones did not. Your feedback also helped me to see that dieters would need some modifications and even some cheats. I'm especially thankful to Andrea Lynn, Nichelle Colley Rothrock, and Stefanie Pascetti who have allowed me to quote them in the book.

If it weren't for nutritionist Leslie Dantchik, the menu plans in this book would resemble the truly boring concoctions I make for myself day after day. Leslie breathed life into this plan by designing menus that were just as mouthwatering as they were quick, easy, satisfying and slimming. Jennifer Iserloh, the Skinny Chef, developed several recipes that undoubtedly will become favorites for many dieters. When I told her that no dieter can live without a martini every now and then, she didn't flinch. Her Orangetini is brilliant.

Finally, I would not be where I am today if it were not for Michael Harriot, my literary agent. Much like Ursula, Michael is a rare gem. Not only does he make sure I get paid top dollar for every word I write, he also serves as my therapist, career coach and friend. I am blessed that he continues to represent me and be a part of my life.

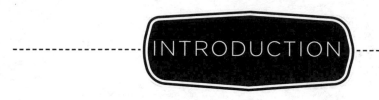

My life used to follow a predictable pattern. Each year, as fall turned into winter, my body slowly but surely expanded. This weight gain often escaped my notice because, among other things, I'm pretty good at that coping mechanism known as denial. Sure, I got on the scale each morning. Yes, I continually saw a higher and higher number. But rather than tell myself, "Oops, I'm gaining weight," I thought any or all of the following:

Must be added muscle from the push-ups I did yesterday.
My hair is longer. Hair weighs something! It must be from that.
I ate a lot of salt yesterday. I must be retaining water.
I ate dinner late yesterday. It must still be in my system and weighing me down. I'll be lighter tomorrow.

There was additional evidence beyond the numbers on the scale. My tummy would begin to sprout a familiar muffin top. I'd pull on my favorite jeans only to find that my thighs didn't quite fit into them anymore. Had they shrunk? Hadn't I told my husband not to put these jeans in the dryer? Hmm. And my face looked a bit rounder. Why was it so puffy? Must be from the wine I had the night before.

Eventually, though, I had to face facts. I usually faced them around February. It was around this time of year when I would barely be able to zip up my knee-high boots. It was tough to come up with an excuse for boots that wouldn't zip. Even I couldn't talk myself into believing my boots had shrunk, too!

This realization often came bundled with depression and lethargy. By midwinter my mood was dark and my thoughts revolved around the following: *Life is exhausting. I don't want to do anything or go anywhere. And now look at me! Now, on top of everything else, I have no clothes that fit. Great. I feel terrible. All I want to do is lie on the couch and have the rest of that creamy pasta. Maybe I'll just finish off that cheesecake. Or maybe both?*

Yeah, it used to get pretty ugly up there in my head toward the end of a long, icy, cold, overcast winter.

Fall and winter were not the only seasons that followed a predictable pattern. As the months got warmer and brighter, I'd spring into dietary panic and nearly starve myself into dizziness and confusion by living on fruit, salads, and sliced cucumbers. By the end of the summer, my jeans and shorts would be almost a size too big! I would pledge to myself that the winter weight gain Was. Not. Going. To. Happen. Again.

(Of course, we all know what happened.)

It was all so frustratingly predictable, not to mention embarrassing. After all, I wrote a health and nutrition column for a newspaper and covered health and fitness topics for various magazines, including *Women's Health*. I'd written about countless diets. At parties, if someone asked about the difference between saturated fat and hydrogenated fat, I could deliver an answer in seconds. In my head, I had a running tally of the calories present in various foods. Eggs? 70. Celery? About 10 per stalk. Bread? Roughly 100 or so per slice, depending on the brand.

If anyone should know how to maintain a healthy weight, I should! Yet I was struggling. At first I thought that I just needed to have more willpower. I thought I needed to practice more self-control. "You just have to eat less," I told myself. "Just eat less."

And believe me, I would try. I attempted to eat less with the sup-port of all of the newest psychological advice around. I had access to all of it. I interviewed the world's top experts on a regular basis and read the various studies as they were released. Still, each winter, the pounds returned.

It wasn't until roughly 2 years ago that I finally realized what was going on. As it turns out, my problem had nothing to do with men-tal softness or a lack of willpower and self-control. After all, I've run marathons! You probably have plenty of self-control and willpower too. Most women do. But if you are like me, and a huge number of other women, you probably also have something else: an incredibly common vitamin deficiency. This vitamin deficiency is fueling your weight gain—especially in the winter—and standing between you and the slimmer, sexier body that you seek.

This nutrient deficiency is widespread and it affects both your weight and your overall health. It's a deficiency in vitamin D, the vitamin that our bodies are supposed to make from sunlight.

As it turned out, every winter—as the days grew shorter—my skin wasn't able to make enough D to supply the cells and tissues with what they needed. Supply fell far short of demand, and my body went into D deficiency. This deficiency made me tired. It caused my muscles to ache and my mood to plummet, both of which eroded my sense of control when sweets were around. And it turned my body into a fat-storage machine.

Then spring and summer would come. Once I was out running and walking in the sunlight, I would naturally build my D levels back up. In the summer, I always had energy, so I exercised more. My mood was better, so I ate less. And my body had the vitamin D it needed to nudge my fat cells out of fat-storage mode and into fat-burning mode. I'm willing to bet that this cycle sounds familiar to you.

Are You Ready to Lose Weight for the Last Time?

I'M SO EXCITED to bring you this plan that optimizes vitamin D—along with several other key nutrients—to help you end the weight gain cycle once and for all. This plan is front-loaded with D and many other powerful slimmers. It helps turn up the heat on your metabolism so you can slim down as quickly as possible.

Perhaps best of all, however, is that once you drop the weight, you'll keep it off. You'll end your battle with winter depression and cravings. You'll be able to drop weight and keep it off year-round. Welcome to the world of lasting weight loss!

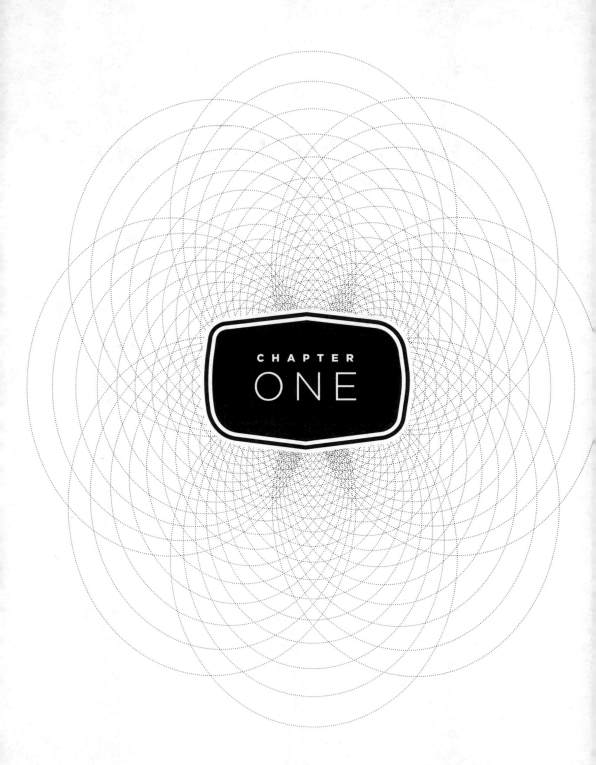

CHAPTER

ONE

Get Ready to Slim Down!

You've probably been told that weight loss takes time—that there's nothing you can do to shrink fat faster. It feels like depressing news, especially at the end of the winter when you realize that—yet again—you've gained the "winter 15," none of your clothes fit, and you now have to focus on extreme dieting just to feel comfortable trying on a bikini before your summer vacation plans.

Good thing most of what you've been told just isn't true!

I've been a health journalist for the past 15 years, and I've covered study after study about diet, fitness, and nutrition. I've interviewed the world's top experts on metabolism, brain chemistry, and appetite. These experts are on the forefront of the science of fat melting, and the research in their labs is starting to turn the common thinking upside down. Based on this massive and growing body of research, we now know that you really can double your weight loss and zero in on your #1 trouble spot—your tummy—while you do it.

Here are a few other surprising things you can do on the 7-Day Slim Down:

➜ **Eat so-called fattening foods.** There's simply no reason to live on egg whites, celery stalks, and chicken breasts. You can and should consume whole eggs, breakfast cereal, bread, dairy, and even cheese. These foods won't give you a bloat baby, send your insulin through the roof, or turn you into a fat-storage machine, either. To the contrary, they are important weapons in your fat-fighting arsenal. That's why they are featured in the 7-Day Slim Down.

➜ **Eat between meals.** Snacking is actually one of the best ways to reduce cravings and stay true to your diet plan. On the 7-Day Slim Down, you have the option of consuming up to two snacks a day.

➜ **Drop pounds without feeling deprived, hungry, or fatigued.** Have you ever experienced Diet-Induced Depression? It feels similar to PMS, and it tends to cause dieters to snap at loved ones over the most minor irritations. It also causes you to feel listless, crave comfort foods, and suffer from foggy thinking.It's completely avoidable if you consume the right nutrients. The 7-Day Slim Down optimizes nutrients that will help to boost your mood as you lose weight—not send you into an emotional tailspin.

➜ **Lose weight without postponing your life.** On this plan, you'll even be able to eat dessert and drink a glass of wine every now and then. There is no one food that is completely off-limits, so you'll never have to cancel a night out just because you're trying to drop pounds. You can follow this plan anywhere—restaurants, holiday parties, you name it.

Why Fat Melting Matters

FOR YEARS, NUTRITIONISTS have been telling us that the weight-loss formula is simple and that it goes like this: eat fewer calories than you burn. Period. And while this is true to some extent, it's also misleading. For instance, this theory has led many people—especially health journalists—to erroneously conclude that eating as little as one extra slice of buttered toast (about 100 extra calories) a day will cause you to gain a whopping 415 pounds over 40 years. This is based on the idea that 1 pound of fat contains 3,500 calories. Thus 100 extra calories a day times 14,600 days equals more than 1.4 million calories, or about 415 pounds.

But this just doesn't happen in real life—whew!

Indeed, the vast majority of people who overeat 100 calories a day gain fewer than 6 pounds in 40 years. That's because as you gain weight, your metabolism increases. So you start burning off some of the extra calories you are eating.

Interestingly, though, some people who consume 100 extra calories a day will gain much more than 6 pounds. Others fewer. How can this be, if they are all overeating the same number of calories? It, in part, has to do with the foods they consume. Certain foods—such as those that are high in protein—take a lot of energy for the body to digest. The stomach and intestines must burn a lot of calories just to break them down. Others, such as foods that are high in fat, take few calories to digest. So 100 calories of protein is actually fewer overall calories in your body than 100 calories of fat.

This is one of the reasons low-carb diets work. But the low-carb lifestyle isn't sustainable for most people, especially women. I'm sure you've tried some version of a low-carb diet and were amazed at the initial results—only to be disappointed when you gained most (if not more!) of that weight back. The food choices on a low- or no-carb diet are just not varied enough to satisfy your taste buds for long, and you end up right back in the vicious weight-loss, weight-gain cycle.

This is not a low-carb diet. Remember earlier, how I said you would be eating bread? Take a peek at the menu plans. You'll see bread, wraps, cereal, and pasta. I don't know about you, but as far as I'm concerned, a diet that doesn't include bread is a diet I don't want to go on! Carbs are a big part of this plan and not just because I love eating them. I've made sure to include them because certain types of carbohydrate foods can actually speed weight loss and help you melt fat faster.

The 7-Day Slim Down, like a low-carb diet, shifts your body into fat-melting mode, but it does it without forcing you to give up the carbs you love! It works by maximizing several key slimming nutrients, the most important of which is vitamin D.

The Hidden Deficiency That's Making You Fat

IF YOU DROP into any health-related discussion board on the Internet, you'll pick up on the buzz quickly. It doesn't matter if the board is focused on sleep issues, fatigue, chronic pain, or stubborn fat. The stories are the same and they go like this:

I struggled with this for years. I went to doctor after doctor and no one could help me. I tried everything! Doctors ran test after test and they couldn't find what was wrong and my symptoms just kept getting worse! Finally I went to a new doctor and, on a whim, she tested my vitamin D level. You would not believe how deficient I was! Now not only have my symptoms gone away, but I'm losing weight, too! It's a miracle!

It sounds like something you'd see on a Saturday morning info-mercial, doesn't it? Yet it's no gimmick. More than 2,000 studies will be published on vitamin D this year alone, making it one of the most researched and most understood vitamins of our time. These studies have convinced experts at prestigious institutions across the world of two powerful truths:

TRUTH #1: Vitamin D deficiency is a worldwide pandemic, one that afflicts the affluent just as much as it afflicts the poor, and one that strikes the fit and healthy just as much as it strikes couch potatoes.

TRUTH #2: Vitamin D deficiency causes, contributes to, or worsens countless diseases and problems, ranging from mood disorders to arthritis to cancer.

And, yes, it contributes to and worsens body weight issues too.

I learned about this common vitamin deficiency a few years ago when an editor at *Women's Health* magazine assigned me to write a story about vitamin D. At that time, I knew little about D, but my editor promised me that it was the new "wonder vitamin." I was quite skeptical—so skeptical that I almost turned down the assignment. I'd been writing and editing health, diet, and nutrition stories for roughly 13 years at that point. During those years I'd seen many "wonder vitamins" come and go. In the late 1990s there was vitamin A and beta-carotene. Then came vitamin E. Resveratrol—the chemical found in red wine—was quite big for a while, too.

For each wonder nutrient, the story was the same. A study would emerge that showed that the nutrient was important for immunity, health, bones, or something else. Then the same nutrient would be touted as the so-called "cure for aging." As coverage built, the nutrient would gain an almost saintly status, eventually earning recognition as the secret cure for everything that could possibly ail a person—including tummy fat.

And then, just when most of society was convinced that it was the cure-all to end all cure-alls, disturbing research would emerge. This research would show that high levels of this nutrient—levels only achievable by overdosing on supplements—worsened cancer or heart disease and increased our risk of death. Eventually enough negative studies would emerge that the nutrient would fall from favor. As a result, over the years, more and more nutrition experts were coming to the following conclusions:

REAL FOODS COME IN A "PACKAGE" THAT SUPPLEMENT MAKERS WILL NEVER BE ABLE TO COPY. Food contains the right balance of nutrients for your body and comes naturally packaged in a way that your body can easily digest, absorb, and use it. Supplements usually come in a package that isn't as easy to digest, absorb, and use. As a result, many of them are never actually absorbed into your body and don't deliver the benefits they should. They go into your body and right back out again.

TAKING TOO MUCH OF ONE NUTRITIONAL SUPPLEMENT WILL CAUSE YOU TO EVENTUALLY BE DEFICIENT IN ANOTHER ONE. High levels of calcium, for instance, block the absorption of iron. Too much soy hinders the absorption of zinc. It goes on and on.

TOO MUCH OF ANYTHING IS JUST AS BAD AS TOO LITTLE OF IT. Experts have warned that taking more than what you need to correct a deficiency can make you just as sick as the deficiency itself. For instance, too much vitamin A or E might increase your risk of cancer rather than decrease it. Too much A can also lead to toxicity: Symptoms include dry, itchy skin; headaches; nausea;

dizziness; blurred vision; and an increased risk of hip fractures. Large doses of vitamin K can damage the liver.

I figured vitamin D would follow the same trajectory. I was wrong.

The Most Studied Nutrient of Our Time

I INTERVIEWED SEVERAL experts for that initial *Woman's Health* story on D, and I grilled those experts quite extensively, asking questions like, "How can one vitamin do so much?" and "We heard the same things about vitamins E and A, and look at what happened with those. Won't we eventually learn that too much D is bad for us, too?"

I wasn't interviewing these researchers and physicians: I was interrogating them. I was skeptical! Yet they patiently answered my questions. My interrogations started with Michael Holick, PhD, MD, of Boston University. Holick had spent his entire career studying the causes and effects of vitamin D deficiency. He'd published hundreds of studies on D, dating all the way back to the 1970s. He believed in the health benefits of D so strongly that he dared to make a controversial recommendation. He promoted "safe sun exposure" so people could get more D from sunlight.

That stance got him fired from the dermatology department at Boston University. He maintained a separate position in the medicine, physiology, and biophysics department of the same university. And even though he was in academic hot water, he didn't back down. If anything, he began working harder to get the word out. (Anyone who is willing to lose their job over something they believe in is someone I want to interview!)

What Dr. Holick told me that day was nothing short of revolutionary. He told me that D—or the sunshine vitamin—was involved in most bodily processes. "There are vitamin D receptors on every tissue and cell in the human body," he said. That means every part of your body—from your brain to your bones to your fat cells—needs D to function properly. As a result, vitamin D deficiency had been shown to cause, trigger, contribute to, or worsen everything from arthritis to cancer to depression to diabetes to osteoporosis. More compelling, however, was that D was not an under-studied vitamin. Thousands of studies had been completed over a span of 40 years, with more and more studies appearing every single day.

At the end of the interview, I thanked him. "I've been writing about health for 13 years," I said. "I've probably written about pretty much everything, at this point. As a result, it's rare to hear something that actually changes my life. But during this 1-hour interview, you've changed my life! I'm going to buy a vitamin D supplement as soon as I hang up the phone."

And I did. I also started to think that the answer was getting more D in my diet, and I began looking into ways to do just that.

How D Helps You Slim Down

ROUGHLY 2 YEARS after I wrote the *Women's Health* article, another magazine hired me to write an article about the link between vitamin D and body fat. Again I was skeptical. For years scientists have searched for a magical ingredient that would help people shed fat. They kept coming up empty. Was D really any more powerful than any other nutrient scientists had studied over the years? The answer is the most exciting weight-loss breakthrough I've ever come across.

As I mentioned earlier, there are vitamin D receptors on our fat cells. This is important because these receptors help to signal the fat cell to either burn or store fat. When D plugs into these receptors, it's a lot like a key that opens a lock. Suddenly, the fat-burning mechanism is unlocked and that stubborn fat that you never thought you would lose begins to shrink.

This mechanism doesn't stop with your fat cells. There are also D receptors in your brain. These receptors need D to keep hunger and cravings in check, as well as to elevate mood.

There are D receptors on your muscle cells, too. This is important because muscle tissue is a robust calorie burner. Each pound of muscle in your body burns 35 to 50 calories a day just to maintain itself. The more muscle you have, the more calories you burn—even while you sleep! Stronger muscles also give you more energy—so you are more likely to burn calories through exercise and everyday movement.

In the winter of 2008, Dr. Shalamar Sibley of the University of Minnesota put 38 obese people on an 11-week diet where they consumed 750 calories less than their estimated daily need. Study participants whose blood levels of D were higher at the study's start lost more weight than participants whose blood levels of D were lower. They actually lost a lot more—70 percent more, to be exact.

By fueling your body with the D-rich nutrients it needs to stay out of a fat-storage state and in a fat-burning state, you can speed weight loss by 70 percent!

The Proof Is Right Here

YOU ARE ABOUT to embark on a revolutionary eating plan, one that was designed by Leslie Dantchick, MS, one of the country's top nutrition experts. It also includes several simple and delicious recipes developed by famed chef Jennifer Iserloh, better known as "the skinny chef." It's based on thousands of studies and interviews with dozens of experts. It's also based on the stunning results of women just like you.

Women's Health magazine also test-drove this plan on dieters before taking this book to press. These dieters had busy lives and real taste buds. They wanted to lose weight, but they didn't want to do it at the expense of the foods they loved. And they wanted to drop those pounds for the last time. Based on their results, you can expect to experience the following:

In just 7 days: You'll feel fuller and more satisfied after eating. Your mood and energy levels will already have improved, and you will have dropped up to 7 pounds.

In 2 weeks: You'll have dropped up to another 2 pounds.

In 4 weeks: You'll be as much as 15 pounds lighter than when you started. You'll also realize that this is the last diet you will ever start.

The rest of your life: You'll maintain a healthy, sexy shape and feel beautiful, happy, and confident—all year long—and while still indulging in the foods you love. It doesn't get any better than this!

The 7-Day Slim Down is a breakthrough program backed by the latest science to help you drop pounds fast. On this plan, you will optimize your consumption of vitamin D and several other slimming nutrients so you can get your body to convert fat into fuel. You'll also:

➔ **Unlock fat burning!** This diet is chock-full of D and other fat-melting nutrients, such as calcium and omega 3 fatty acids. These nutrients work synergistically to help you drop pounds fast. All of the cells in your body house receptors for vitamin D, including your fat cells. When there's enough D throughout your body, the vitamin is able to plug itself into the receptors on fat cells. When it does this, it's like a key that turns a lock, allowing fat cells to release calories to be burned for energy. Adequate D also optimizes the absorption of calcium, another important weight-loss nutrient. Calcium promotes weight loss by binding to fat in your gastrointestinal (GI) tract, preventing some of it from getting absorbed into the bloodstream, and, like D, it also promotes fat burning.

➜ **Zero in on your #1 trouble spot!** Studies show that dieters who maximize D and other featured nutrients on this plan don't just lose weight twice as fast, they lose it where they most want to lose it—their tummies.

➜ **Blast through plateaus!** Usually when you go on a diet, your weight loss slows as your body shrinks. That's because your metabolism adjusts as your body gets smaller, causing you to burn fewer calories. This, of course, makes it harder and harder to lose weight with each pound you lose. This is why so many people hit a stubborn plateau long before they've reached their goal. The 7-Day Slim Down helps you avoid plateaus by fueling you with nature's most potent fat-melting foods and nutrients—foods that preserve muscle mass, turn up the heat on metabolism, and encourage your body to incinerate fat.

➜ **Wake up happy!** I don't know about you, but my past attempts at dieting have made me feel irritable and downright angry at times. Again, D comes to the rescue! Like fat cells, the brain also has D receptors—here, D boosts levels of serotonin. This mood-elevating chemical helps you feel good, especially during the winter months, so you can gain a sense of control and stay motivated. Most winter "comfort food" cravings come from your body's attempt to self-medicate and temporarily boost serotonin levels. Unlike simple sugars that result in a short-term mood boost—one that is often followed by rebound depression and overeating—D boosts your mood and energy levels all year long.

➜ **End your battle with hunger!** The 7-Day Slim Down is front-loaded with foods that release satiety hormones early in the digestive process, allowing you to automatically fill up on fewer calories. This diet is also rich in nutrients like soluble fiber that slow the transit of food in the small intestine, keeping satiety hormones elevated for a longer period of time after you eat. This means that you are less likely to feel hungry between meals. By maximizing your consumption of satisfying foods, the D diet minimizes the hunger and cravings that cause so many dieters to call it quits so early in the diet.

→ **Boost your health and add years to your life!** Don't you hate that nagging, fear-inducing question, "I may get skinny on this diet, but at what cost to my health?" I hate that too. I also hate when a diet makes my face feel greasy, upsets my stomach, and generally makes me feel stressed out, hungry, and weak. On this plan, you'll shed pounds quickly, and you'll also reduce your risk for cancer, diabetes, depression—even the common cold. And the nutrient-rich foods on this plan are designed to work with even the most sensitive stomachs and dietary needs.

Seven Reasons to Start This Plan—Today

I PROMISE: YOU are going to fall in love with this diet just as you've probably fallen hard for Ryan Gosling. But unlike Ryan Gosling, this diet will love you back! Here's why.

1 **No foods are off-limits.** This is not a low-anything diet. You can and will continue to consume the healthful fats that you love—including guacamole, olive oil, and whole eggs. You can also continue to savor a glass of wine at night, if that's your pleasure. And dessert is always on the menu if you want it!

2 **You get to eat carbs.** Go ahead and wave good-bye to low-carb deprivation. By normalizing levels of D, you'll be able to consume reasonable amounts of carbs and still lose weight. That's because D helps normalize insulin levels. When you're insulin sensitive, eating food sends glucose into your cells, satisfying you and lowering hunger hormones. But if you are not insulin sensitive (read: insulin resistant), glucose can't enter muscle cells as easily for use as fuel. So this excess circulating glucose that can't get inside your muscles indirectly triggers hunger hormones and you eat more, make more fat, and eventually gain weight. D keeps you insulin sensitive so hunger stays in check.

3 You won't have to live on tiny portions. In addition to D, The 7-Day Slim Down plan is also packed with high-volume, low-calorie foods that will fill you up on fewer calories. Plus when D plugs into receptors on fat cells, the cells secrete the hormone leptin, which travels to the brain and communicates the "we're full, so just stop eating" message. When there's not enough D to plug into these receptors, not as much leptin gets released and you feel hungry when you should really feel full.

4 You don't have to do military style work-outs. Leave the pull-ups, push-ups, and pain to women who enjoy torturing their bodies. On this plan, you'll choose from several different movement options that will fit into your day and lifestyle. But, perhaps more importantly, the eating plan works synergistically with the fitness plan. By optimizing D, you'll be more likely to feel like moving in the first place. Low D can make you feel achy and tired, making you want to rest on the couch and blow off your workouts.

5 You don't have to give up your social life to get skinny. You can eat out on this plan and

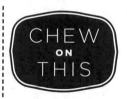

CHEW
ON
THIS

A study by Atascadero State Hospital in Atascadero, California, found that athletic performance improved when D levels were brought up to optimal levels.

you can also drink wine and indulge in dessert. You'll never feel as if you can't go out with friends just because you are on a diet.

6 **You don't have to be rich to afford it.** On this plan, there's no fasting, cleansing, or juicing required. It's also not based on any magical, expensive, or hard-to-find ingredients. It's a sensible, yet delicious diet that any woman can follow and enjoy for a lifetime.

7 **Even vegetarians can try it.** I'm a vegetarian, too, and I designed this plan to be easily customized for anyone's dietary needs. Many of the featured foods on this plan come from plants. They include orange juice, mushrooms, and tofu. Nonvegan vegetarians can also look to eggs and dairy to help them melt fat. And pescatarians can shed fat with salmon, oysters, and more.

Frequently Asked Questions

HERE ARE SOME things you might be wondering about the 4-Week Slim Down.

Q: Can I drink alcohol?

A Yes! Just count it as one of your snacks. You may have one glass of wine or one beer a day on this plan. You'll even find a great martini recipe (called the "Orangetini) in the recipe section. It's great for Girls' Night.

Q: If I find myself getting hungry between meals, what can I do to help me feel full longer?

A Make sure you are consuming all of the recommended foods! This is a plan that shouldn't leave you hungry. Make sure you're actually eating the two snacks I recommend each day.

Also, shift your meals earlier, consuming lunch around 11 or 11:30 a.m. and dinner around 5:30 or 6 p.m. If you are still hungry, you can load up on unlimited raw vegetables.

*Q: **Do I have to do the workouts outlined in Chapter 14, or can I use my own?***

A   If you already have a workout schedule that works for you, by all means, stick to it. The exercises outlined in this book are simply meant to get you moving and boost your metabolism—feel free to use whatever fitness method does the same for you already. Get bonus weight-loss points for doing some of that activity outdoors. Just make sure to *always* wear sunscreen on your face and never keep your body in the sun for more than 15 minutes without sunscreen.

*Q: **I'm a vegetarian. Can I still follow this plan?***

A   Yes, you can. Many of the star foods on this plan are vegetarian options, including dairy, tofu, and mushrooms. I've worked hard to include several vegetarian options in the menus and recipes. If you'd like to try a different recipe that features fish or meat, just swap the same amount of tofu for the fish or meat.

*Q: **Can I eat out on the plan?***

A   Yes, you can. I don't recommend you eat out a lot during week 1, though.

Your first week on the plan is an important one. It's a time when you want to focus all of your energy on getting used to the diet.

After that, it's perfectly okay to eat out occasionally. Many of your 7-Day Slim Down, Winter Menu, and Summer Menu options are easily found at restaurants. I've marked these as great eat-out options. For many of them, I've also provided advice on how to modify the selections when you're at a restaurant. You can find special eating-out advice, along with dozens of suggested menu options, in the Appendix.

Q: **What happens if I really screw up?**

A Say, one night, you eat a bag of microwave popcorn followed by half of a chocolate cake. It happens, and it happens to the best of us.

There's no need to be perfect on this plan. In fact, perfection is not recommended. Women who try to follow their diets perfectly are the ones most likely to fail—or, at least, to feel like they've failed. That's because the black-and-white thinking of "I'm on a diet" is too rigid. Everyone needs a special treat or indulgence every now and then. That's why I recommend the 90/10 principle—as long as you eat the right foods 90 percent of the time, you can afford to "cheat" the other 10 percent. You certainly shouldn't overdo it every meal of every day, but consciously allowing yourself a treat once a week or so will not derail you. In fact, that treat will help you stick to the plan and continue losing weight.

The reality of overeating is that it takes a *lot* to gain a noticeable amount of weight. It takes 3,500 calories of overeating to gain just 1 pound. That's the number of calories in 3 quarts of full-fat ice cream! The next time you feel you've overdone it, remind yourself that it's not as bad as you think and just get right back on the plan. You're more in danger of gaining weight by snacking too much over time than by consuming too much food in one sitting. So remember: 90/10. What you eat most of the time is what really matters.

No matter how big your indiscretion, get in the habit of always recommitting to the diet. Don't start dieting again tomorrow. Start today. Start right now. Start this second. Learn from your mistakes rather than obsessing over them.

How to Use This Book

IN THE MANY years I've written about diet and nutrition, I've learned that there are two types of dieters. Some just want the menu plans. They don't care how and why the diet works—they just want to get started! Then there's the other type of dieter. That's the person who's tried everything and yet nothing has worked. This is the kind of woman who wants proof, studies, science, and testimonials.

Depending on which category you fall into, you'll want to use this book differently. If you just want the menus, then go ahead and skip what I've listed below as "optional." On the other hand, if you are the kind of woman who wants and needs proof, you've got it! Whether you start at the beginning or flip back and forth, you'll find plenty of fascinating information, studies, and real-life stories to back up the plan.

Here's a quick preview of the rest of the book so you can gain a sense of what you want to take the time to digest and what you can safely skim or skip.

OPTIONAL READING

CHAPTERS 2 THROUGH 6: These chapters offer the science and support for this plan. This is where you'll find all the evidence you need, including biological, anthropological, biochemical, hormonal, and nutritional support for D and weight loss. And it's fascinating stuff! You'll learn not only how this diet's star player—vitamin D—boosts health and helps you shed fat faster, but also how this one vitamin may just be the solution to most of our ills.

REQUIRED READING

CHAPTERS 7 AND 8: In these chapters you'll get all the background you need on how to follow the diet. You'll also take a simple test that will help you determine whether you are D deficient. Like most women, you probably are, but take the test anyway. It will help you understand how vitamin D works and determine whether you need a supplement, when you need it, and how much you should take.

THE DIET STARTS HERE

CHAPTERS 9 THROUGH 12: In these chapters, you'll find several diet plans ranging from a quick, 1-week Slim Down designed to help you drop pounds fast to a winter diet chock-full of warming, hearty foods that satisfy.

THE 7-DAY SLIM DOWN (CHAPTER 9)—This is a 1-week jump start designed to help you drop pounds fast. You can either start the diet here or go straight to Chapter 10, if you prefer a less-intense approach.

THE 4-WEEK SLIM DOWN (CHAPTER 10)—You'll follow these menus no matter what season you initially go on the diet, and you can mix in options from Chapters 11 and 12, depending on the season.

THE WINTER WARMING MENUS (CHAPTER 11)—These are winter menus, with foods designed to warm the soul. These recipes and meals seriously satisfy and help prevent cravings. These menus are also higher in D during the months when you need it most.

THE SUMMER LIGHT MENUS (CHAPTER 12)—These are lighter, cooler meal options—perfect for those hot summer months. They are also slightly lower in D because you'll be getting some of the vitamin from sunlight.

THE SUPPORT YOU ABSOLUTELY NEED

CHAPTERS 13 THROUGH APPENDIX: In these final chapters, you will find what you need to stay true to the plan and experience lasting results. I've included 37 delicious, quick, and easy recipes to help you get slim and stay that way. Many of these recipes were developed by Jennifer Iserloh, also known as "the skinny chef." Jennifer is the author of *Secrets of a Skinny Chef* and has developed recipes for Jessica Seinfeld and Joy Bauer, the nutrition consultant for the *Today* show. She is known for her rich, yet slimming, meals. I'm so thankful she agreed to create recipes for this plan! When you make and taste her recipes, you will be thankful, too.

In the remaining chapters, you'll find exercise routines that help tone and define, as well as lists of recommended brands, tips for eating out, and much more. You'll find everything you need to follow this plan for life—because I want this to be the last diet you ever start. I want you to love this diet, and in turn, love your new body. I want you to experience real success. I want you to lose weight and keep it off—for the rest of your life!

And I want you to do it while you enjoy every single bite of the food on your plate.

Let's do this.

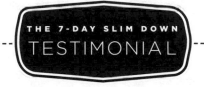

"I lost 7 pounds on the first week of this diet, and my husband lost 4! In the past, I've been my own worst enemy with dieting. With school and work, I rarely have had time to cook and often eat out. With the 7-Day Slim Down, I prepare most of the food I need on the previous day. I have yet to find a recipe that I do not like. It keeps me full throughout the day. I definitely recommend it because there is nothing difficult about it. It's a great diet. It's just so simple."

—STEFANIE PASCETTI, 24, COLORADO SPRINGS, CO

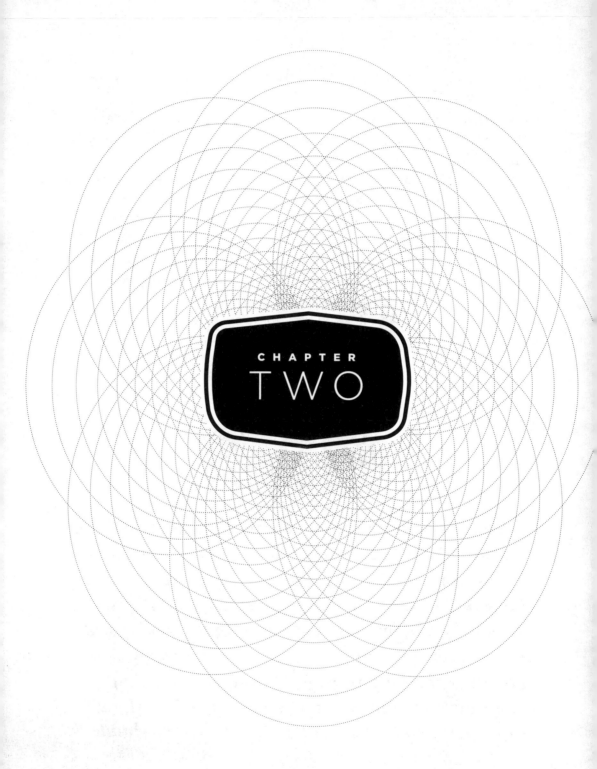

CHAPTER
TWO

The Slimming Magic of Vitamin D

As you will learn in the coming chapters, getting enough D in your diet is critical to helping you melt fat, boost your metabolism, reduce your appetite, reduce the frequency and intensity of your cravings, and feel energetic enough to exercise and enjoy life. And yes, it will help you shed that muffin top for good!

As I mentioned in Chapter 1, if you just want to skip to the diet plan, please do! But if you're curious—or even skeptical—about how this diet works and why, keep reading. This diet is based on 90 years' worth of combined research and tens of thousands of studies. The evidence in support of D is anthropological, historical, biochemical, and statistical. It all comes together here to help you lose weight and feel better than ever.

To help you fully understand just how important D is for your waistline and overall health, I'd like to take you on a brief journey through time. This journey starts millions of years ago. It continues through the caveman and hunter-gatherer era and progresses to the 1800s, 1900s, and eventually to the new millennium and today. Ready? Let's go.

The Birth of Today's Wonder Vitamin

LET'S TRAVEL BACK millions of years, to a time when humans didn't yet inhabit the Earth. Nearly all of the world's living beings still lived in the oceans, where they bathed in, drank, and breathed a calcium-rich fluid that helped them form their skeletons.

Eventually some of these early creatures crept out of the oceans and onto dry land. On land, the need for a strong skeleton was greater, but they were no longer surrounded by calcium. So they adapted. These early land creatures developed the ability to produce an important nutrient in their skin, and that nutrient allowed them to make a small amount of calcium go a very long way. With the help of sunlight, the cholesterol in their skin converted into vitamin D, which then entered their bloodstream. The D allowed these early land creatures to absorb more calcium from the scant amounts found in the foods they consumed. This way, they got enough calcium to fuel all of the many electrical interactions in their bodies as well as strengthen their bones. Without this development, land creatures would have remained flimsy with soft bones—much like fish. They would not have been able to absorb enough calcium to survive.

Now fast-forward a couple hundred million years. Humans first entered the picture somewhere in Africa near the equator. These humans had very dark, melanin-rich skin. (Melanin is a pigment that gives skin, hair, and eyes their color. It also absorbs heat and UV radiation from the sun, protecting skin from burns and cancer.) Early humans needed this protection because they spent most of their days outdoors, either gathering food or hunting for it. Sure, there was no hole in the ozone layer back then and sunlight wasn't quite as intense and damaging as it is today. But these early humans spent many more hours in the sun than we do today. The dark melanin-rich pigments in their skin helped them to avoid blistering sunburns. Their bodies adapted to high doses of D, and that vitamin became necessary to the proper functioning of every cell and tissue.

Then these humans did what humans seem to do best—they paired off, procreated, and made more humans! As the population grew, humans migrated farther and farther away from the equator. But in these regions north and south of

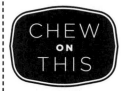

CHEW
ON
THIS

Because early humans spent so much time in the sun, their bodies were able to make 20,000 IU or more of D a day.

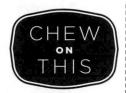

the equator, the days grew shorter and the sun grew less intense. Now the melanin in their skin was problematic because it was filtering out too much sunlight. Some of these hunters and gatherers—especially the ones with the darkest skin tones—were having trouble making enough D from sunlight to support their skeletons.

As a result, the humans with the darkest skin became weak. Their bones grew brittle and they suffered many health problems. Some died during childbirth and many young D-deficient children died before adulthood. Consequently, vitamin D deficiency created a natural selection that caused skin color to evolve to become lighter and lighter. The farther north these humans migrated, the lighter their skin color became. In climates in the far north, lighter skin still wasn't enough to ensure humans got enough D. These humans adapted by harvesting vitamin D–rich fish, which enabled them to live in dark, northern climates like Alaska and Scandinavia.

So far, so good. Evolution and the survival of the fittest allowed humans to make no matter where they decided to live. Everything went along swimmingly for thousands of years (at least in terms of their vitamin D levels, that is).

And then came the industrial revolution. From the 1700s through the early 1900s, people began leaving rural farm life and going to work in factories. That was when a strange and puzzling disease called rickets began to develop. Rickets caused bones to remain soft and flimsy, like the cartilage in fish. In young children, gravity molded these overly soft bones into deformities—bowed legs, knock-knees, and spinal misalignment. These children also suffered other debilitating symptoms: painful spasms, difficulty breathing, convulsions, nausea, and even death.

Initially, scientists and physicians were perplexed. They thought that, as with many other diseases of the time, poor hygiene might be the culprit. Some, however, thought that rickets, like scurvy, might be the result of a nutritional deficiency. These experts thought that the adults and children who got rickets just weren't eating enough fresh vegetables. Other experts, however, blamed the disease on a lack of fresh air. Still others thought it developed from lack of exercise.

Oddly, rickets seemed to disproportionately affect children who lived in urban areas. It took many years, but eventually scientists began to realize that city living was mainly dark and devoid of sunlight. People worked indoors. Children played indoors. Even when people were outdoors, buildings and smog blocked sunlight. Adults and children on farms, however, outdoors for much of the day, suffered far fewer cases of rickets.

Could it be, scientists wondered, that sunlight was essential for good health? Back then scientists did not know what they know now. They didn't know that a cholesterol-like substance in the skin (called 7-dehydrocholesterol) transforms into a precursor of vitamin D when it is bathed in ultraviolet light. This precursor is eventually transformed into active D through the help of the liver and kidneys. Back then, scientists didn't know about D at all. It hadn't even been discovered or named.

For this reason, they did not know precisely why sunlight might help cure rickets. They just suspected that it could. Other pieces of evidence seemed to confirm this hypothesis. For instance, the disease was much more rampant in people with darker skin colors—skin that blocked more sun rays. Scientists also noticed that rickets tended to worsen during the winter months and nearly disappear in the summer, when sunlight was more prevalent.

Soon a cure for rickets was born: sunlight. Physicians began exposing babies to the sun for 15 minutes to an hour a day. It worked! They called it heliotherapy, a therapy that would later be used to treat various other diseases including depression and various skin conditions (like psoriasis).

Around this time, a scientist named Sir Edward Mellanby was experimenting with different diets and seeing how they affected dogs that he happened to be raising and keeping indoors, without access to sunlight. The lack of sunlight was not intentional, it was merely convenient. Still, Mellanby discovered that feeding the dogs porridge (which is naturally devoid of D) induced rickets, whereas feeding them cod liver oil (which happens to be rich in D) cured it.

Thus, in addition to sunlight, cod liver oil became a standard treatment and prevention for rickets. Soon parents were forcing children to down 1 to 3 teaspoons of the stuff a day. Today, fish oil comes in convenient, time-release capsules that are flavorless, and liquid fish oil is often infused with orange, lemon and other flavors to improve its taste. Back then, however, it was another story entirely. (My mother has told me stories of her own mother chasing her and her brother around their New York apartment, trying to get them to swallow the vile stuff. It smelled foul and tasted oily—the kind of oily that you can't get out of your mouth once you get it in.)

Initially, scientists didn't know why cod liver oil or sunlight worked. One theory was that cod liver oil was rich in vitamin A, which had already been shown to cure another debilitating disease: beriberi. It wasn't until another researcher did a similar experiment with cod liver oil lacking A that vitamin D was discovered and named. Soon food manufacturers were irradiating milk, bread, and other foods with ultraviolet light to produce D. Once these D-fortified foods hit the marketplace, rickets disappeared in the United States.

Not a Vitamin at All

IN THE 1960s, 70s, and 80s, true appreciation for D began to grow. Over the years, researchers realized that vitamin D was not actually a vitamin at all. Technically speaking, a vitamin is a vital substance that the body cannot make on its own. But, unlike other vitamins, the body can make D.

And this D acts more like a hormone. In other words, D has more in common with the sex hormones estrogen and progesterone and the stress hormone cortisol than it has in common with vitamins A, C, and E.

Researchers also realized that D might be more powerful and more important than just some substance that seems to prevent rickets. This realization began to surface in the late 1960s when Anthony W. Norman, PhD, at the University of California, Riverside and researchers at the University of Wisconsin and the University of Cambridge in England were all working to figure out the chemical structure of D and trace its journey through the body from skin to blood to liver to kidneys to cells.

Norman discovered that cells in the intestines had receptors for D. When D plugged into these receptors—much as a key fits into a lock—it allowed more calcium to be absorbed into the bloodstream. It was a monumental discovery.

Researchers already knew that calcium was an important mineral, one that was needed to build and maintain healthy bones. Calcium was also known to be important for the proper functioning of blood vessels, muscles, nerves, and cells. If D helped calcium get into the bloodstream, a person with a D deficiency would probably also develop a calcium deficiency—thus worsening the health of all of these bodily systems and tissues. In this roundabout way, a D deficiency could harm everything from bone health to the proper functioning of electrical signals among cells in the brain and elsewhere.

Over the years, researchers discovered that D did even more. In addition to helping the intestines absorb calcium, it also served as a signal that told bones to absorb calcium or to release it when it was needed elsewhere in the body.

At first, however, it seemed as if calcium was the star and D was merely a supporting player—almost like calcium's bodyguard. Eventually, however, experts began to see that it was actually the other way around. D seemed to be involved with much more than just calcium regulation. In the coming decades, Norman and many other researchers discovered more and more D receptors. They weren't just in the intestines. They were also in the brain, in the

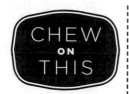

heart, in hair follicles, on muscle cells, in bone marrow, on immune cells, in cancer cells, and, yes, even in fat cells.

Researchers were able to find D receptors on nearly every cell, organ, and tissue in the body. D, as it turned out, was even important for gene regulation, an important finding when it came to the prevention of cancer.

An increasing number of scientists now believe that D may affect diseases and disorders as disparate as colon cancer, multiple sclerosis, premenstrual syndrome, psoriasis, high blood pressure, depression, and more. Here's a look at just some of the findings.

CANCER: When researchers added D to cancer cells, the cells stopped maturing and growing. A 2008 study found that women who had a vitamin D deficiency when they were diagnosed with breast cancer were 94 percent more likely to have their cancer spread than women with adequate levels of vitamin D.

AUTOIMMUNE DISORDERS: Rats fed D had less inflammation and less overly aggressive immune responses when wounded or burned, showing that D might help to control overactive immune response in autoimmune diseases. In a different study, a topical version of D was used to control psoriasis, an autoimmune disease in the skin.

BODY WEIGHT: University of Michigan researchers found that D-deficient children tended to gain more fat over 30 months than children with normal levels of vitamin D.

LONGEVITY: People are more likely to die in the winter, when sunlight is less intense and our levels of D are lower.

IMMUNITY: Vitamin D plays an additional important role in promoting the production of cathelicidin, an effective defender against fungal, bacterial, and viral infections, including the common flu.

MOOD: Vitamin D deficiency has also been shown to contribute to depression. Activated vitamin D in the adrenal glands helps regulate an enzyme necessary for the production of dopamine, epinephrine, and norepinephrine—the hormones critical to mood, stress management, and energy.

MEMORY AND ATTENTION: Vitamin D appears to have extraordinary, positive effects on the brain. One study found that middle-aged and older men with higher levels of vitamin D were more mentally agile and consistently performed better in tests of attention and information processing.

BLOOD SUGAR CONTROL: Vitamin D deficiency also impairs insulin production and increases insulin resistance.

Indeed—vitamin D has become one of the most studied "vitamins" of our time.

I interviewed Dr. Norman in the summer of 2011. He told me that, back in 1969, he was just one of a few people who were studying D. Another was Michael Holick, PhD, MD, a professor at Boston University. You'll be hearing a lot from and about Dr. Holick and Dr. Norman in this book because

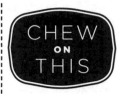

Studies show that vitamin D decreases:

- *Your risk of cancer by 30 to 50 percent.*
- *Your risk of developing type 2 diabetes by 55 percent.*
- *Your risk of developing multiple sclerosis by half.*
- *Your risk of getting heart disease by 33 percent.*

they've both made important contributions to the current understanding of D's role in the body.

Since those early days, interest in vitamin D has soared. Along the way, Dr. Norman has made a hobby of counting the number of studies that are published on D each year.

▸ In the 1970s, there were only 150 studies published on vitamin D each year.
▸ In 2005, this shot up to 1,500.
▸ In 2010, more than 2,000 studies were completed on D.
▸ In 2011, it was up to 3,000.

Indeed, the research is robust and it's convincing. D deficiency has also been linked to Crohn's disease, rheumatoid arthritis, high blood pressure, thinning of the bones, joint and muscle pain, and depression. It can even raise your risk of getting dementia and Parkinson's. Experts now believe that D deficiency might trigger or worsen just about any illness or disease you could possibly name. But on the plus side, if you replenish your D supply, you'll be a much healthier—and fitter—person.

Clearly, this is not one of those understudied fads. The importance of vitamin D is here to stay.

More Than Weight Loss

NOW, I KNOW you picked up this book because you want to lose weight, and not necessarily because you want to beat cancer or strengthen your bones (although those are certainly added benefits). In the next few chapters, you'll find all of the evidence about D and body weight that you will ever need or want. You'll find studies and information about how D helps you slim down faster. And you'll learn how it also reduces hunger and fuels you with more energy.

For now, however, I want to mention something that I think is incredibly important. It's this: Because this diet optimizes D— along with several other key nutrients—it will do more than help you slim down. It will also help boost your well-being and even extend your life.

I've been on a lot of diets—probably more than the average woman. If a magazine hires me to write about a particular diet, I don't just interview experts about it. I go on the diet myself. By test-driving the diets I write about, I am able to ask better questions, write better articles, and develop stronger programs. Not to mention I'm always up for losing a couple of pounds!

So, I can tell you something with great conviction: It's not fun to be on a diet that isn't good for your overall health. I'll admit that I've experienced this personally. Constipation? Not fun. Fuzzy-forgetful brain? Not fun. Greasy skin? Not fun! The shakes? Seriously, not fun.

In my opinion, any diet that slims you down at the expense of your health and well-being isn't worth the trouble. Do you really want to lose weight at the expense of your heart? How about your bone health, or your mood? Is it really worth it to lose a lot of weight but suffer from depression, develop osteoporosis, or experience constipation or migraines?

I can't answer those questions for you, but I hope the answer is no. It's not worth it, and it's also not necessary. You can drop pounds without frustrating, even dangerous side effects. You really can.

The 7-Day Slim Down will help you lose the weight, but it will also help you get in the best shape of your life—physically, mentally, and emotionally.

The Deficiency Strikes Back

NOW LET'S GET back to that history lesson for a bit. When I left off, we'd just finished the industrial revolution and rickets had been cured by the food fortification program. You might be

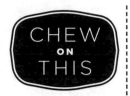

The number of rickets cases doubled between 2002 and 2003 and the disease began making an appearance around the globe—in Canada, New Zealand, the United Kingdom, the United States, Australia, Ethiopia, and Saudi Arabia.

wondering, "If fortified foods have eradicated D deficiency, then why is this diet even necessary?"

Here's why: You're not getting all the D you need. You might be getting enough to prevent rickets, but you're not getting enough to fuel weight loss and overall good health. Yes, it's rare for any well-fed American to be severely deficient in any vitamin or mineral, and fortification solved the problem of D deficiency for many years. But by the turn of the millennium, something strange began to happen. Rickets began making a comeback.

As it turns out, D deficiency is growing. More and more people being tested are deficient. The National Health and Nutrition Examination Survey (NHANES) found that only 23 percent of teens and adults had a sufficient amount of this essential vitamin in their blood. That percentage was nearly half that amount in a similar study done a decade before. In some populations, vitamin D deficiency affects 82 percent of people.

What exactly is going on? No one knows for sure, but here are a few of the leading theories.

▶ With television and computer games replacing outdoor play, children spend less time outdoors than ever before.
▶ When children and adults are outdoors, they wear sunscreen, which blocks the creation of D in the skin.
▶ Fewer people are drinking milk, the leading delivery system for fortified D.
▶ Adults are working longer and longer hours and two or more jobs, spending more time indoors and away from sunlight.

Because it takes a severe D deficiency for rickets to develop, the disease is still relatively rare. However, other diseases that might be caused or triggered by D deficiency are not rare at all. These include various autoimmune diseases such as rheumatoid arthritis and psoriasis, various cancers (even skin cancer!), osteoporosis, and, yes, obesity.

Are You Really Deficient?

IT'S IMPORTANT TO note that, while vitamin and mineral deficiencies are common throughout the world, they are not as common in the United States. Deficiencies tend to be widespread in low-income and drought-ridden countries in Africa and Southeast Asia, and they tend to disproportionately affect young children, pregnant women, and people who are so skinny that their main goal is to gain weight, not lose it. In such places, vitamin A deficiency is so extreme that 250,000 children go blind from it each year, with half of them dying from the deficiency.

In the United States, though, food is overly plentiful. Even though few Americans eat the recommended number of vegetables, most are extremely well fed and well nourished. It's rare for an American to be deficient in any vitamin or mineral. But D is one exception to that rule.

According to the National Health and Nutrition Examination Surveys published in the *Archives of Internal Medicine*, 77 percent of Americans are D deficient. The deficiency numbers get even higher among minorities, whose darker skin pigmentation makes it more difficult to generate vitamin D: 90 percent of Hispanics and 97 percent of African-Americans have insufficient blood levels of vitamin D, which may also account for higher rates of obesity in these populations.

And even in warm, sunny states, people are not immune. In a study of young women in Los Angeles, where sunlight is as prevalent as breast implants, 25 percent were seriously deficient in D and 59 percent were suboptimal.

It's tempting, of course, to look at those statistics and think, "I'm probably in the 23 percent who gets enough D." I know this because that's what I thought about myself. It wasn't until I began consuming a D-rich diet—one much like the diet you'll find in this book—that I realized how deficient I must have been.

Can Too Much D Make You Sick?

THERE ARE TWO types of vitamins: water-soluble vitamins and fat-soluble ones. Water soluble vitamins dissolve in water and easily travel through the various watery fluids of your body, such as your blood. Because of this, they don't spend a lot of time in your body. They are either quickly used or discarded. If you take too much of a water-soluble vitamin, you'll end up with one thing: expensive urine.

Fat-soluble vitamins are stored in your fat. That means they stick around for a while and, unlike water-soluble vitamins, can build up in your body. Taking too much of one of these can be toxic. Toxic isn't good. Toxic makes you sick and can even kill you if you don't address it. Vitamin D is fat-soluble. For years, experts have been cautioning against taking too much of it for just that reason. They worried high amounts could be toxic.

Then, in the spring of 2010, a well-known health and nutrition guru named Gary Null became extremely ill. He suffered excruciating fatigue and pain as well as kidney damage. Eventually a physician was able to diagnose the cause: Null was suffering from vitamin D toxicity.

As it turned out, Null was accidentally consuming more than 1,000 times more D than he'd thought he was getting 2,000 IU. In reality, he was consuming 2 million IU. It was all due to a faulty supplement (his own brand, actually), which was 1,000 times more potent than it was supposed to be. The supplement was soon pulled from the shelves and Null sued the manufacturer that bottled the supplement.

So, it's true—someone did get sick. And the media initially jumped on this story and used it to "prove" the dangers of taking too much D. But the media missed a crucial element of this story. Gary Null was only able to consume that much D by accident. It was an isolated fluke due to a manufacturing problem. Had his supplement not been faulty, he would never have gone toxic. He would have had to take 1,000 pills a day to reach those toxic levels!

In reality, it's extremely difficult to induce vitamin D toxicity. That's why there are so few cases of it. Physicians have been dosing their severely deficient patients with 10,000 IU of D daily for 6 months, without any toxic effects. That's 16 times the Institute of Medicine's vitamin D recommendation. Think about that. Doctors are giving patients a dose that is 16 times higher than recommended and no one is getting hurt. You would have to take at least five over-the-counter supplements to reach the medically prescribed dose that physicians use to correct severe deficiency. That's a lot.

The amount of D that I recommend in this book is only one-fifth the amount physicians give their severely deficient patients. It's the amount that physicians, researchers, and dietitians told me they take every single day. It's also the amount I take as a supplement, in addition to consuming a diet (the very one recommended in this book) that is also high in D. In reality, toxicity—or D overload—is just plain rare. It's also easily reversible. On the other hand, D deficiency is much, much more common.

Why Not Just Go Outside?

BUT, YOU MIGHT wonder, why do you need D from food or supplements at all? Why can't you just get more sun?

Ideally, you would get your D from the sun. After all, that's what our hunter-gatherer ancestors did, and it's what our bodies are genetically designed to do. When your skin makes its own vitamin D, the vitamin lasts twice as long in your blood as when you eat the vitamin or get it through a supplement. But there are several problems with getting all or most of your D from the sun. They are both obvious and not so obvious.

THE RISK OF CANCER AND WRINKLES. Even if you had the time to hang out at the beach every day in your favorite bikini, any sunscreen you slather on is going to block D. Sunscreen reduces your skin's ability to make D by 90 to 99 percent, depending on the SPF. And as any dermatologist or magazine will tell you: Sunscreen is the key to beautiful skin as you age. Without it, you not only increase your risk of wrinkles, but of skin cancer, too.

INCONVENIENCE. Even if you weren't into skin protection and didn't mind looking weathered and old before your time, you still wouldn't be able to get enough D because your skin rarely connects with the sun rays needed to trigger the production of D. There are many days during the winter months when we see little to no sunlight at all. There are other days when we are only outdoors in the morning or late afternoon, when the sun's angle is too oblique to trigger the production of D in the skin. And when we are outdoors, we don't have enough skin exposed. Your face alone can't make enough D in 15 to 30 minutes to satisfy your body's needs. You need to expose a larger surface

SUPPLEMENTS

Supplements are a good idea. I take a D supplement, and I recommend you take one, too. But supplements are not a replacement for a healthy, D-rich diet. This, in part, is because many experts believe most of us need even more D than the typical 2,000 IU supplement provides, so eating D-rich foods helps to boost your numbers. It's also because food delivers benefits and comes in a package that the smartest nutrient manufacturers have never been able to copy.

   The 7-Day Slim Down *is a complete nutrition and health plan that makes the most of dietary sources. I've done all the research and found the best, most delicious sources of D. For example, sun-dried shiitake mushrooms have a whopping 1,600 IU of vitamin D—almost your entire daily allowance. Don't love shrooms? That's okay. I'll show you how to combine satisfying dairy (an 8-ounce glass of fortified milk has but 100 IU) with fish, eggs, margarine, and other foods to maximize your D intake and fuel your weight loss. Fortified products such as tofu, yogurt, OJ, almond and soy milk, bread, and breakfast cereal are all great options, too.*

area—your arms, your back, your legs. Few of us wear clothing that allows us to do that during the middle of the day.

AIR POLLUTION. Smog can filter out some of the UVB rays, so less of them are able to reach your skin. This is one reason why folks who live in Los Angeles and Atlanta tend to be deficient despite their sunny, warm locations. Another might be that, in hotter climates, people are more likely to stay indoors with the AC on and to routinely use sunscreen.

GEOGRAPHIC LOCATION AND TIME OF YEAR. If you live further north than Atlanta, you essentially can't make any vitamin D from November through March because the angle of the sun isn't correct. The sun is too low in the sky for enough rays to penetrate the atmosphere and make their way to your skin. You also spend a good portion of this time of year indoors. And, chances are, when you are outside, it's dark.

The Right Amount of D

AN INSTITUTE OF Medicine report released in November of 2010 recommended that Americans should get 600 IU daily of vitamin D, up from 200 IU (the level set in 1997). The panel also raised the acceptable upper limit of daily intake to 4,000 IU for adults, up from 2,000.

But the Endocrine Society has a much higher recommendation and so do many other experts. Why such varying numbers?

In part, the differences are due to confusion over the optimal blood levels of D. The Institute of Medicine based its recommendation on blood levels of 20 ng/ml, as that level seems to be where the bone-building benefits start. But other experts recommend more—in the neighborhood of 40 to 60 ng/ml, because all of the other health benefits have been shown to take place when blood levels are that high.

While you can probably get blood levels to 20 ng/ml on a diet that only consists of 600 IU of D—without a supplement and without sun exposure—you cannot get to the higher amounts without a supplement or at least some sun exposure.

"The Institute of Medicine is extremely cautious," Dr. Norman told me. "Their guidelines are based on what they think is good for bone health, but that doesn't address what's needed to benefit your immune system, pancreas, muscles, heart muscle, and brain."

Dr. Norman and others told me that the optimal daily D dose for weight-loss and other health benefits is 1,000 to 2,000 IU of supplemented D, plus a D-rich diet, plus safe sun exposure.

And that's exactly what this plan recommends and provides.

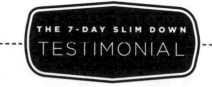

THE 7-DAY SLIM DOWN
TESTIMONIAL

"I've gained and lost 5 pounds over and over again for the past 5 years. Last year I started exercising and I firmed up, but the scale didn't move much. I started the 7-Day Slim Down because I wanted to lose weight so I'd have more energy to do sports activities with my family. After reading the menus, I was very excited to get started. After 1 week, I lost 1.5 lbs! The recipes and menus are very easy to follow. There are no crazy ingredients that you don't have at home already. My favorite recipe was the Chicken Scallopini with Garlic Mushroom Sauce, actually my family loved it, too! I would definitely (and have) recommend this diet to anyone who gains weight in the winter and is looking for an easy to follow plan,"

—NICHELLE COLLEY ROTHROCK, 41, HOCKESSIN, DE

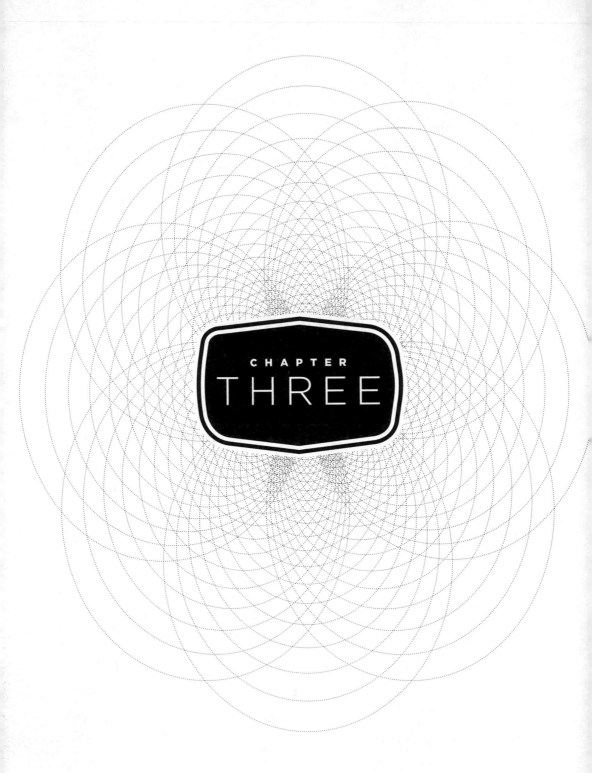

CHAPTER
THREE

How You'll Slim Down

Many women tell me that they practically have to starve themselves to lose any weight. They eat unbelievably small portions, skip meals, or live on shakes and meal replacements. Yet this drastic calorie cutting seems to shrink only a few pounds off their frames.

Of course, no one can maintain such a strict food existence. All it takes is one night out with friends. One glass of wine leads to another and then to a plate of nachos drenched in glow-in-the-dark cheese—and before you know it, you're waking up with a food hangover. It's a slippery downward slope that often leads to watching the numbers rise on the scale instead of sending them in other direction.

In two words: "Been there."

Starvation-style dieting always fails because it's impossible to follow for very long. It intensifies hunger and cravings. It also slows your metabolism, putting you on an impossible quest to eat smaller and smaller portions to keep the weight loss going. No matter how motivated you might have been at the onset of a starvation-style diet, you always end up in the same place. It's a total bummer.

It may sound obvious, but too many women still don't believe it: Starvation isn't a prerequisite to a smaller body. Neither are liquid diets, carb-free diets, or other types of deprivation diets. You can lose weight without starving yourself or drastically restricting your food choices. You can eat reasonable portions and put in reasonable workouts at the gym, and you can shed fat while you do it.

It all comes down to eating the right combination of foods— foods that will shift your body out of fat-storage mode and into fat-melting mode. Specific vitamins and nutrients can actually help to flip an internal switch that signals cells throughout your body to burn more calories, wasting many of those calories as heat. Without these important nutrients, the opposite happens. Your body holds onto fat. Your metabolism slows and your weight-loss efforts become an exercise in futility.

The 7-Day Slim Down optimizes these critical slimming nutrients so you can finally drop those stubborn pounds and keep them off for good. In this way, you can still consume reasonable portions and put in a reasonable amount of exercise. Yes, you still have to watch your portions. Yes, exercise is still important. But fat-melting foods work in your favor so you can eat and move in a way that is reasonable, effective, and realistic for life.

Your Internal Fat Switch

WE TEND TO think of our fat cells as ugly storage units and, to some degree, that's exactly what they are. They are capable of keeping us alive in emergency situations—for example, if you were to find yourself stuck at the North Pole without provisions your fat cells could literally save your life. A 150-pound woman has well over 100,000 calories stored in her fat cells—enough energy to keep her going for a month or longer without a single bite of food. I bet you wouldn't think of your fat cells as "ugly" after that!

Back in the day when food was scarce, these fatty storage units were quite handy. It was a lucky cave gal who could get fat just looking at an antelope and whose body clung to fat no matter how long she subsisted on blueberries and twigs. And it was this lucky cave gal—the one who gained weight easily and lost weight slowly—who tended to remain fertile and pass on her easy-gaining genetics, especially during hard times.

As a result, most of us non-cave-dwelling women now have some of the easy-gaining cave gal's genes. We have fat cells that easily and effectively absorb fatty acids and glucose from our blood, converting them into fat to be stored until later.

Unlike that cave gal, though, most of us never have a "later" when we need that stored fat. Food is always plentiful, so unless we go on a diet, the fat keeps going into storage and never coming back out. The 7-Day Slim Down helps reverse fat accumulation and switch on fat melting in three important ways.

FAT-MELTING TACTIC #1:

CELLS BURN CALORIES WHEN INSULIN TELLS THEM TO

Our fat cells secrete a number of proteins and hormones that travel to the brain, liver, muscles, and other organs. In fact, your fat cells probably make more hormones than any other organ in your body— even your ovaries. These hormones influence what and how much fat your muscles can burn. They tell your liver and other organs when to start making more fat to be stored. They influence when and how much you eat. They affect blood clotting. They even govern whether or not you can get pregnant.

Most of these hormonal signals are tied closely to insulin sensitivity. Insulin is a hormone secreted from your pancreas. One of its jobs is to help glucose get into body cells, which burn glucose for energy. How well insulin pushes glucose into cells is called "insulin sensitivity." The more sensitive your cells are to insulin, the better. The less sensitive they are to insulin, the more likely the calories you eat will end up in your fat cells.

If you've been on any type of diet during the past decade, then you've probably heard of insulin sensitivity. Low-carb diets touted it as the reason that carbs were evil. While insulin sensitivity is very important, there are other ways to achieve it beyond banning carbs completely from your diet. (Can I already hear a sigh of relief?)

Low-carb diets boost insulin sensitivity by reducing insulin's workload. When there's less glucose, there's less for insulin to do, so blood levels of insulin stay low. This makes cells more likely to notice and respond when insulin levels do rise.

The 7-Day Slim Down makes your cells more sensitive to insulin through a different, much more delicious mechanism—and one that is more realistic, long term. It does this by normalizing your levels of vitamin D. Study after study shows that this vitamin helps to ensure body cells listen and respond to insulin. For instance, an Iranian study published in the *American Journal of Clinical Nutrition* found that consumption of a daily yogurt drink fortified with 500 IU of D twice a day for 12 weeks (for a daily total of 1,000 IU) led to a marked improvement in blood sugar and insulin levels for study participants with type 2 diabetes, compared to a study group that did not get D in their yogurt.

FAT-MELTING TACTIC #2:

FAT CELLS RELEASE CALORIES TO BE BURNED RATHER THAN HOARD THEM IN STORAGE

As I've said, scientists have discovered vitamin D receptors on many cells and tissues throughout the human body. A receptor is a molecule that is found on the surface of a cell. When vitamin D attaches to a D receptor, it acts like a key opening a lock. This, in turn, triggers a number of actions to take place within the cell, including:

▶ The fat cell becomes more metabolically active and burns more calories.
▶ The production of cortisol—a stress hormone that encourages the formation of stored belly fat—decreases.

When levels of D are low, levels of parathyroid hormone (PTH) rise. Higher than normal levels of PTH trigger a series of reactions that eventually lead to fat cells converting sugar into fat and hoarding fat rather than releasing it to be burned, explains Michael B. Zemel, PhD, director of the Nutrition Institute at the University of Tennessee in Knoxville. A Norwegian study of 3,447 men found that elevated PTH levels increased their risk of becoming overweight by a whopping 50 percent.

When D isn't plugged into receptors, it can interfere with leptin signaling. Leptin is an important hormone that signals your brain to

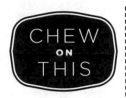

stop eating. A lack of vitamin D may interfere with this appetite-suppressing hormone. Your body doesn't know when it's full, so you continue to eat.

FAT-MELTING TACTIC #3:

MUSCLES INCINERATE FAT TO POWER EVERY MOVEMENT

We can't have much of a discussion about fat burning without talking about muscle tissue. Your muscle cells act like a furnace for the human body. Every pound of muscle burns 35 or more calories a day just to maintain itself, and it burns even more as it powers every movement you make.

Your muscles are capable of burning many types of fuel. They can burn fat (ideal), and they can also burn protein (not ideal) and carbs (which may or may not be ideal, depending on the circumstance). Let's start with the carbs. Your muscles store 500 to 1,000 grams of carbohydrate (in the form of glycogen). Although that sounds like a lot, it's really only about 2,000 to 4,000 calories. Your body is capable of burning through all of that stored energy during a day of fasting or during endurance exercise, such as a marathon.

Ideally, you want your muscles to burn very little of this stored carbohydrate. That's because dropping muscle glycogen stores trigger hunger. The hungrier you get, the more likely it is that you'll overeat. This is why The 7-Day Slim Down encourages your body to preserve glycogen while preferentially burning fat. It does this by optimizing vitamin D, as well as calcium.

In addition to the carbohydrate I just mentioned, your muscles are also composed of protein. When you go on a diet, your muscles usually burn a combination of fat and protein. Ideally, you want to increase the fat burning and decrease the protein burning because it's the protein that keeps muscles strong and your metabolism humming along. The more protein your muscles cannibalize during a diet, the slower your metabolism and the harder it is for you to maintain your results.

The 7-Day Slim Down helps you preserve muscle protein and preferentially melt fat, again by dosing you with optimal amounts of vitamin D and calcium, specifically from dairy products. Research from McMaster University in Canada has found that women who consumed dairy products as a part of their weight-loss regimen were able to lose only fat and completely preserve muscle. They also lost the fat where they wanted to lose it—their tummies. "And the participants gained muscle mass, which is a major change in body composition," explained Andrea Josse, lead author of the study and a graduate student in the department of kinesiology at McMaster University. "The preservation of muscle is very important for maintaining metabolic rate and preventing weight regain, which can be a major problem for many seeking to lose weight."

Muscle is also important in helping to create a long, lean physique and in making your skinny jeans look fantastic on you. So the more muscle you can preserve and create, the better!

Why You Gain Weight Every Winter

DO YOU REMEMBER those early humans that I mentioned in Chapter 1? They were hunter-gatherers who lived in Africa, spent all day outside, and as a result, adapted by maintaining very high levels of D in their bodies.

And when those early humans eventually migrated north, they developed the ability to store D in their fat in order to survive the long, dark, northern winters. Each summer they spent hours and hours outdoors, exposed their skin to lots of sunlight and produced lots of D. Since food was plentiful, they also plumped up during the summer months. This extra fat served as storage rooms for D, much as our bones serve as a storage room for calcium and other minerals.

Back then, being able to store D in your fat was a seriously good trait to have. Humans who could plump up during the summer, both with excess fat and excess D, had a much greater chance of surviving the long, cold winters when food—berries, seeds, and even wild animals—was harder to come by.

Now let's fast forward to today. Our bodies still store D during the sunnier summer months. During this time of the year, our skin soaks up sunlight and makes more D than our cells and bloodstream need, storing the excess in our fat.

Our bodies do this to ensure that we have enough D to make it through the winter. But our bodies can only access that D if we lose weight (much like our ancestors would do from a lack of available food). Recent research shows that it takes a drop of 15 percent of your total body weight before enough D is released from the fat to do you any good. For a 200-pound woman, that's 30 pounds. How many 200-pound women do you know who drop 30 pounds every winter due to food scarcity?

Not too many, right?

Here's why: Winters are no longer lean times for most of us. We're surrounded by more calories in the winter than we are in the summer! We're stuck indoors with a fridge full of cheese, a freezer full of ice cream, and cabinets full of snack chips. Worse, we're invited to holiday parties, social events, and work functions where delicious sweets and fried little morsels are passed around on pretty serving trays.

So instead of getting leaner during the winter, we do the opposite: We get fatter.

As a result, our D remains in storage and we go into deficiency. It's already hard enough to remain lean during the winter, what with all of the culinary temptations I just mentioned. But when D levels dip into deficiency, it leads to more problems: depression, muscle aches and fatigue, fat storage, overeating, and weight gain.

Why Haven't You Heard about D until Now?

SO YOU MIGHT be wondering, "If D does all of this, how come I've never heard of it before?"

There's a good reason for that. As I mentioned in earlier chapters, nutrition experts have been burned time and time again when their studies seemed to show the promise of a particular vitamin, the vitamin became a fad, and then subsequent studies proved the vitamin was not a miracle cure.

After the rise and fall of vitamins A, E, and beta-carotene, among many others, the scientific community got extremely cautious. Even as support for D built over the years, few people made a fuss. Rather, they hesitated, saying more research was needed. And, for many years, it really was.

Scientists had noticed an association between D and body weight for years. Various studies, for instance, had shown that people who weigh less tend to have higher 25 (OH)D (25-hydroxyvitamin D) levels. People who weigh more have lower levels.

Yet experts assumed that association was just that: an association. The scientific method states that an association is not the same thing as causation. For instance, the murder rate is associated with ice cream consumption. That association could falsely lead you to believe that ice cream consumption is causing the murder rate to go up. People eat ice cream and the next thing you know, they are pulling out AK-47s and shooting people. Time to ban ice cream, right? Nope. Just because two things are associated with one another doesn't mean one causes the other.

Experts initially thought that D was associated with body weight, but that it didn't necessarily impact it. They figured that the two were probably interrelated by another mechanism. Being over-weight raises your risk for a number of health problems, ranging from heart disease to diabetes to cancer. For years, experts thought that vitamin D deficiency was just one more problem that was caused by obesity. And there's some solid evidence to show that this is indeed the case: Obesity does seem to cause D deficiency.

One way obesity seems to cause D deficiency is what I like to call the Hotel California Effect. Fat stores D much like this: D can check in, but it can't easily check back out anytime it wants. Because of the Hotel California Effect, it takes 50 percent more D to bring blood levels up to normal in the obese than it does in the lean. The obese also make roughly 57 percent less D when they are exposed to sunlight than the lean do.

"The chemical structure of D is such that it prefers to sit in a layer of fat rather than hang out in a watery substance like blood," explains Dr. Norman. In other words, the fatter someone becomes, the more D gets trapped in their fat cells and the less D is available to circulate in the bloodstream and get to the cells that need it. In this sense, obesity can cause vitamin D deficiency. But can vitamin D deficiency also cause obesity?

As it turns out, it can. The evidence didn't start to emerge until just a few years ago.

That's when Shalamar Sibley, MD, did what was supposed to be a routine study at the University of Minnesota. With 100 men and women, it was a small study by research standards. Yet it was the perfect size for what Dr. Sibley wanted to investigate: how weight loss affected blood pressure regulation.

It wasn't the kind of study that earns a researcher national attention, but then, on a hunch, Dr. Sibley decided to run one more test. It was for vitamin D status.

"In the research I noticed building support for the idea that vitamin

D had effects on fat metabolism," Dr. Sibley told me. "I wondered, 'What if someone's vitamin D status could impact their ability to succeed at weight loss?' We were already running this study anyway. I figured I might as well test their vitamin D status, too."

The results were startling.

Participants with adequate blood levels of vitamin D lost more weight than participants with suboptimal levels—even though everyone was consuming the same number of calories. For every increase of 1 ng/ml in the level of 25-hydroxycholecalciferol—the precursor form of vitamin D—study participants lost one-half pound more.

At around the same time, researchers in Norway looked at the diets and lifestyle factors of 9,252 men and 9,662 women. They studied the association of everything from coffee consumption to smoking to vitamin D intake and how it all related to body weight. The more vitamin D people consumed, the less they weighed. It's important to note that this study was done in a country that is very far north and has days of total darkness during the winter months; in Norway, vitamin D deficiency is rampant. People who consumed the least D tended to be the heaviest.

Several other studies added the missing pieces to the causation puzzle, and now, in just the past couple of years, more and more researchers and organizations have come on board and agreed that D deficiency and excess fat work together to create a vicious cycle, each worsening the other.

"It's a circular problem," says Dr. Norman. "D deficiency can set you up to gain weight, and gaining weight can set you up for D deficiency."

The cycle can start as early as conception. An Indian study, for instance, found that babies born to D-deficient moms grew up to have less muscle mass (which can lower metabolism) and more insulin resistance (which causes everything from overeating to fat storage) compared to children born to moms with normal D levels. And a University of Michigan study found that D-deficient children tended to gain more fat over 30 months than children with adequate levels of D did.

Here is more research to consider.

▶ When humans migrate from high-altitude living—where sunlight is stronger and D deficiency is lower—to a low altitude—where sunlight is weaker and D deficiency is stronger—they tend to gain weight.

▶ People also tend to gain weight in the winter (when D levels are lower) than in the summer.

▶ People also tend to be fatter in northern climates, where D levels are lower.

▶ A Norwegian study of 3,447 men linked diets low in vitamin D with elevated fat storage hormones and a higher risk of obesity.

▶ A McGill University study linked low D levels with increased levels of muscle fat, a problem that weakens muscles.

The Supporting Body Slimmers

NOW D IS pretty incredible and effective, but it's not the only player on this slimming team. If it were, this would be just another fad diet. As you may already know, fad diets usually involve one star food or ingredient, which the entire diet is based around. On these diets you might be eating enormous amounts of grapefruit or acai berries or some other "magic" ingredient. Such plans conveniently overlook the fact that no woman can live on one food or one food group for the rest of her life.

I don't believe in fad diets. I believe in diets that work. As I've said, this diet is different. This is not about losing weight just for bikini season. It's about losing weight for bikini season (or whatever reason applies) and keeping it off forever.

If D were the only slimmer on this plan, you just wouldn't be able to follow the diet because you'd have to eat one ingredient—like salmon—every single day. I don't know about you, but I can't eat salmon every single day for the rest of my life! And if I can't do something, I'm not about to ask you to do it, either.

That's why the 7-Day Slim Down includes several additional body slimmers. It's the combination of these slimmers that allows you to eat a variety of foods and still turn up your metabolism and melt body fat. Here's a quick rundown of each of them and why they are so important.

Calcium

HOW IT SLIMS: Calcium is a mineral that works in tandem with D to help you shed fat. Calcium is stored in fat cells, and researchers think that the more calcium a fat cell has, the more fat that cell will release to be burned. Calcium also promotes weight loss by binding to fat in your GI tract, preventing some of it from getting absorbed into your bloodstream.

Research done by Dr. Zemel at the University of Tennessee and many others shows that people who follow a high-calcium diet lose more fat from their bellies than people who consume a low-calcium, reduced-calorie diet. One of Dr. Zemel's studies, for instance, found that dieters who consumed 1,100 milligrams (mg) of calcium daily (from three daily servings of yogurt) lost up to 22 percent more weight and 61 percent more fat than dieters who ingested less calcium but who consumed the same number of calories.

When researchers at Creighton University surveyed many different studies, they found that higher calcium intake was correlated with lower body weight. Each 300-mg increase of calcium resulted in 2.2 fewer gained pounds in children and 5.5 to 6.6 fewer gained pounds in adults. In another study, published in the *British Journal of Nutrition*, obese women who were put on a 15-week diet and took 1,200 mg of calcium lost six times more weight than women on the diet alone.

The research on calcium and body weight is so vast and convincing that, for many years, calcium stole the show and gained nearly all of the research attention, not only when it came to weight loss, but also when it came to strong bones. As it turns out, however, you could take megadoses of calcium and see almost no results if you are deficient in D. That's because D enables your body to absorb calcium from the food you eat. A person who is vitamin D–deficient will absorb only one-third as much calcium as she would with a healthy vitamin D status.

But the two seem to work together in other ways that aren't completely understood. When dieters consume optimal amounts of D and calcium, they lose more weight than dieters who don't boost their consumption of these nutrients. And other research finds that not only do you lose more, you are also less likely to regain what you drop.

"When you get enough D and calcium, you'll boost the effectiveness of your dietary and exercise program by up to 70 percent," says Dr. Zemel. That's an extra quarter pound of fat every week!

Protein

HOW IT SLIMS: While this is not a low-carb, high-protein diet by any stretch of the imagination, the 7-Day Slim Down does include a source of protein at every meal. In addition to keeping hunger in check, these regular doses of protein help to keep body composition—the amount of fat relative to muscle—in better proportion. Along with calcium and D, protein helps you to preserve muscle mass as you drop pounds. A recent study out of the University of Illinois found that women who consumed protein twice daily lost 3.9 percent more weight than women who consumed less of it on a diet. They not only lost more weight, they also got stronger as they did so, with their thigh muscles alone ending up with 5.8 percent more protein at the end of the diet than before.

"We believe it's important to eat protein in the morning and through the day so those amino acids are always available," says Mina Mojtahedi, a researcher on the study. "Unfortunately, American women tend not to eat much protein, especially when they're trying to cut calories."

Omega-3 Fatty Acids

HOW IT SLIMS: You almost can't consume D without consuming omega-3 fatty acids, and that's a good thing. Fatty fish like salmon (which are also high in D) are one of the richest sources of this fat. Other foods, such as some nuts and seeds, contain a type of fat that can be converted into omega-3s after ingestion.

Omega-3s enable weight loss by switching on enzymes that trigger fat-burning in cells. They also help to boost mood, which may help reduce emotional eating. And omega 3s might improve leptin signaling in the brain, causing the brain to turn up fat burning and turn down appetite.

In one study done in Iceland, participants lost 2.2 more pounds over 4 weeks when they supplemented with fish oil or ate more fatty fish like salmon, compared to participants who did not supplement or consume fatty fish. In a French study of 27 women with type 2 diabetes, 3 grams of fish oil daily (the amount in roughly 6 ounces of salmon) reduced body fat levels by 3.5 percent and abdominal fat by 6 percent, even though study participants did not change their eating or exercise habits.

Monounsaturated Fatty Acids (MUFAs)

HOW THEY SLIM: MUFAs are a type of fat found in olive oil, nuts, seeds, avocados, peanut butter, and chocolate, and they have just one chemical bond (which is why they are called "mono" unsaturated).

Although the 7-Day Slim Down isn't necessarily loaded with MUFAs, I've made sure to feature some foods with high levels of MUFAs because they are important for metabolism. One Danish study of 26 men and women found that a diet that included 20 percent of its calories from MUFAs improved 24-hour calorie burning by 0.1 percent and fat burning by 0.04 percent after 6 months. Other research shows that MUFAs zero in on belly fat. Specific foods that are high in MUFAs—especially peanuts, tree nuts, and olive oil—have been shown to keep blood sugar steady and reduce appetite, too.

MUFAs are also good for your overall health. Plus many high MUFA foods—such as guacamole—are what make my life worth living. I figured you might feel the same. That's why I've made sure to include high MUFA foods like chocolate, peanut butter, and guacamole as options on the plan.

Conjugated Linoleic Acid (CLA)

HOW IT SLIMS: CLAs are potent fat burners that are found, along with D and calcium, in dairy products. They are fatty acids that are created when bacteria ferments the food in the first part of the stomach of cows, sheep, and other ruminant animals. The CLA that is created through fermentation then makes its way into the meat and milk of these animals.

When we consume these foods, the CLA helps blood glucose enter body cells, so CLA can be burned for energy and not stored as fat. CLA also helps to promote fat burning, especially in muscles, where the bulk of our calorie burning takes place.

In an Ohio State University study of 35 women, study participants who took 8 grams (g) of CLA daily lost more weight, especially from fat, than women who took a placebo supplement that did not contain CLA. And in a University of Wisconsin study of 23 people who took 4 g of CLA daily, participants burned more fat—even while asleep—than participants who took a placebo. Finally, a study of 118 men and women in Norway found that those who took 3.4 g of CLA each day lost 3 percent more body fat over 6 months than participants who took a placebo.

Now, there's a downside to this slimmer. Most of these studies involved huge amounts of CLA—amounts that you'd only be able to consume if you ate 40 pounds of beef at once. I don't know about you, but I certainly can't eat 40 pounds of beef for dinner, no matter how hungry I am!

That doesn't mean CLA is worthless, though. You might not be able to consume enough of it through food alone to melt off a huge amount of fat, but you can consume enough of it to help nudge your metabolism into a fat-burning state. And when you add it to the other slimmers on the plan—especially the D, calcium, and protein—you will create the perfect environment for total-body fat burning.

Optional Slimmers

I'VE MADE THE following slimmers optional on the plan because many people just plain don't like them. I highly recommend you incorporate them if you're up for it, but they are not required. If you'd like to speed your results, by all means, use and enjoy them! If not, don't worry; you'll still lose weight swiftly.

Capsaicin

HOW IT SLIMS: Capsaicin is the chemical that makes hot peppers taste hot in our mouths. It activates receptors on heat-sensing neurons on the tongue—and in the gut. And it's the activation of the neurons in the gut that's so important for fat burning. When these neurons get turned on, they stimulate your body to produce heat. That's why you feel hot and sweaty after you eat hot peppers. And this heat production burns calories.

In a University of Maryland study of 80 overweight men and women, participants who took 6 milligrams of capsaicin a day for 12 weeks lost more abdominal fat than those who took a placebo. Although total weight loss was similar between the groups, those who took the capsaicin burned more fat and preserved more muscle mass. Remember: More muscle equals more calorie burning.

The hotter a pepper tastes, the more capsaicin it contains. But please don't force yourself to eat these foods if you can't stand them. There are enough fat burners on this plan to get you to your weight-loss goal without suffering through one spicy meal after another. For those of you who love jalapeños and other hot foods, definitely feel free to kick it up a notch. Doing so will get you to your goal more quickly.

Polyphenols

HOW THEY SLIM: Polyphenols are the antioxidants that give green tea its health- and metabolism-boosting punch. Research shows they boost resting metabolic rate by up to a whopping

17 percent, helping the body to burn more fat. One recent study done on rats found that EGCG, the polyphenol in green tea, blocked weight gain and prevented metabolic syndrome when rats were fed a high-fat diet. You can actually feel this effect after you drink the tea. Your body will literally heat up as your cells waste calories as heat. Green tea is a great winter elixir for that reason. Drink a cup whenever you feel chilled and are tempted to eat even though you are not really that hungry. The tea will warm and soothe you, reducing hunger and cravings.

THE WHOLE SLIMMING PICTURE

Now before you start superdosing yourself with all of these slimmers and waiting for the fat to magically melt away, let's be clear: D and other slimmers facilitate weight loss, but they are not magic pills. If you just took a bunch of supplements, you might see some effect—for instance, by swapping some fat for muscle. But you wouldn't see the dramatic results I'm promising on this plan.

To see serious weight loss, you'll need to combine these slimmers with portion control. The menus in *The 7-Day Slim Down* do just that. They help you to optimize all of the slimmers mentioned in this chapter, as well as hold you to about 1,400 daily calories—without having to count them yourself. When you do both, you can expect to speed your weight loss by as much as 70 percent.

The best part is that you'll be able to do it without feeling excessively hungry or suffering from the intense cravings that may have derailed other diet attempts in the past. To find out how the 7-Day Slim Down keeps appetite and cravings in check, just turn the page.

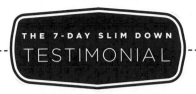

"I gained about 10 pounds since going to culinary school about 6 years ago and trying to get it off just wasn't working out so well. I tried straight-up calorie counting through an app on my phone. I contemplated other programs. I eventually tried the 7-Day Slim Down plan. When I started the 7-Day Slim Down, I wanted to lose those 10 pounds so I could fit into my wedding dress. This diet helped me do just that. I dropped $2\frac{1}{2}$ pounds the first week and about 1 pound a week after that. Even though I've reached my goal, there are certain things that I will always incorporate into my eating habits. Like the hard-cooked eggs as snacks—brilliant! They filled me up as a quick snack, and my fridge is always stocked with them now. Also, the almond and orange juice was another snack that I loved. Before the 7-Day Slim Down, I tended to opt for egg whites, thinking that whole eggs were too indulgent. Now I've learned to use whole scrambled eggs for a filling breakfast. I also really enjoyed the Sardine and Egg Sandwich for lunch. Again, it was easy and very much filled me up. Sometimes I couldn't even eat the whole sandwich in one sitting, which is shocking because I can down food."

—ANDREA LYNN, 33, ASTORIA, NY

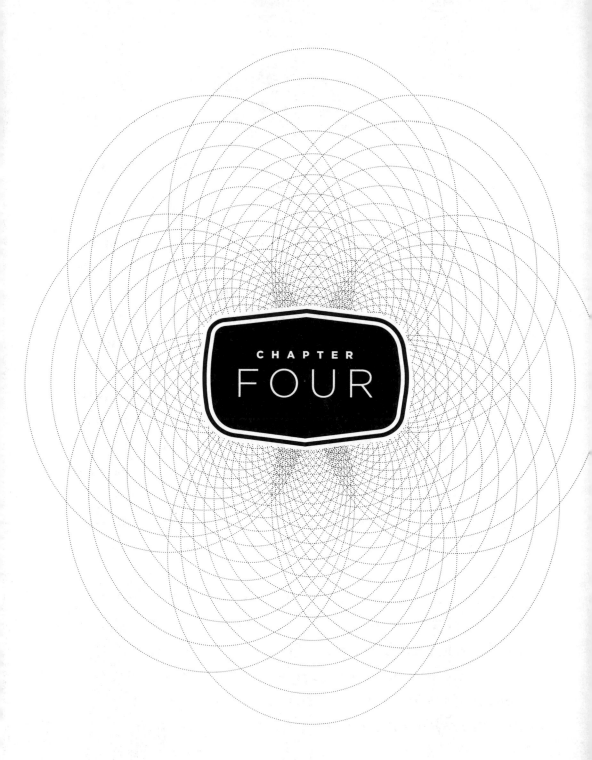

CHAPTER

FOUR

How You'll Beat Hunger

I'm sure you've been on a diet before, finished a serving of food, and thought, "Really? I'm supposed to feel satisfied on that? They have got to be joking."

It's not a fun experience is it?

I'll tell you what else isn't fun. It's that moment during the middle of the afternoon when you start to get that gnawing sensation in your stomach. You look at the clock and realize your next meal isn't supposed to happen for hours. But hunger is already setting in, and it's setting in in a big way. You're supposed to be concentrating on important stuff—like that presentation you are putting together or the to-do list you're writing. Yet your brain feels like it has been replaced with cotton. All you can think about is how hungry you are and the giant bag of chips you're going to rip open as soon as you get home.

Do I even need to describe how tense and grumpy this can make you feel?

It's for all of these reasons and more that I knew the 7-Day Slim Down needed to do more than help you drop pounds fast. It had to fill you up, too. After all, who can stick with a diet that leaves them feeling hungry, confused, light-headed, and grumpy all the time? I definitely can't. So in addition to building vitamin D and several other slimmers into this plan, I've also made sure to build in a number of important nutrients that will help you feel satisfied, reduce hunger between meals, and ward off diet-induced depression. On the following pages, you'll find out how it all works.

The Science of Appetite

TO UNDERSTAND HOW this plan helps you turn down hunger, you need to understand why you feel hungry in the first place. It all starts in your head.

Your brain acts a lot like a computerized fuel gauge that directs you to fill up whenever it notices that its gas tank (your stomach) is empty. Your brain responds to many different messages that come from all over your body. It gets messages from nerves that surround your stomach. It receives messages from various hormones, too. These hormones come from your stomach, your intestines, your pancreas, and your fat cells. Some hormones communicate "empty." Others communicate "full." When many "empty" messages come in at once, the brain turns up appetite and turns down metabolism. When many "full" messages come in at once, it turns down appetite and turns up metabolism.

Remember: Our bodies are designed to help us survive famines. So as soon as we start dieting and we lose a few pounds, hunger hormones rise—causing us to feel even hungrier. Have you ever noticed this about 3 or 4 weeks into a diet? Everything will be going well. You've lost 5 or more pounds. Then, wham! Suddenly food starts looking better. It starts smelling better. It starts tasting better. That's actually your brain's survival mechanism at work.

The 7-Day Slim Down overrides this evolutionary mechanism by feeding your body ultrasatisfying foods—foods that flip every single fullness switch in the body. To see this in action, let's take a hypothetical journey through the body. We'll compare a typical meal from The 4-Week Slim Down with two "quick fix" options that you might reach for to satisfy a craving. Let's see how the following options affect your hunger differently:

OPTION #1:	OPTION #2:	OPTION #3:
The 4-Week Slim Down's Tuna Tacos	Meal replacement shake (aka Dieter's Old Standby)	Pint of ice cream followed by bag of potato chips (aka The PMS Dinner)

Ready to compare?

Tuna Tacos: They Keep You Satisfied

IN YOUR MOUTH: Tacos are crunchy and messy, which helps satisfy your oral yearning for texture. Tacos are also a slow eating adventure. They require a bit of chewing, and they tend to get your hands a little dirty. All of this works in your favor because the more time you spend with food in your mouth, the more satisfied you will feel after you've eaten. This also buys your stomach and intestines time to communicate the "I'm full" message to your brain.

IN YOUR STOMACH: The avocado in the taco is loaded with fiber. There's additional fiber in the corn taco shell and various fillings. This fiber makes the taco relatively heavy and bulky, and once it all mixes with other liquids in your digestive tract, it expands and becomes even heavier.

As a result, it doesn't take too many bites of taco to weigh down and blow up the stomach like a water balloon. This puts pressure on nearby nerves (called stretch receptors). These nerves act like landlines that connect the stomach to the brain. Although there are many different nerves capable of transmitting messages from the stomach to the brain, one large and important one is called the vagus nerve. Think of it like the Bat phone.

As the stomach puts pressure on the vagus nerve, this nerve tells the brain, "We're full," and then the brain flips an internal switch that turns off your sensations of hunger. In addition to high-fiber foods, heavy, water-filled foods—such as most fruits and vegetables—are also very filling. They weigh down the stomach, filling you up on fewer calories. The 7-Day Slim Down features optimal amounts of both high-fiber foods and heavy, water-filled foods so you can fill up on fewer calories.

IN YOUR BLOODSTREAM: The fiber from the avocado and the protein from the tuna both slow transit time in the intestine. That means that the taco sits around for a while and breaks down very slowly. This slow digestion provides a long and steady amount of food energy to the bloodstream. Slow increases in blood sugar help to shut off hunger and keep it off. Quick increases tend to cause a rebound effect. You feel satisfied for a bit, but then hunger quickly returns with a vengeance.

This rebound effect is caused by the hormone insulin. If you've ever been on a low-carb diet, then you've heard of insulin. This hormone signals cells throughout the body to take up glucose and burn it for energy. But when blood sugar rises quickly, the pancreas sends out a lot of insulin at once. This drives sugar out of the bloodstream and into cells all over the body—including fat cells. Once sugar drops in the bloodstream, hunger returns.

The taco also keeps you satisfied for another reason: It's high in D. Several studies have linked low levels of D with disruptions in insulin and blood sugar, leading to both type 1 and type 2 diabetes. D helps make you insulin sensitive. When you're insulin sensitive, eating food shuttles glucose into your cells, satisfying you and lowering hunger hormones. But if you are not insulin sensitive (read: insulin resistant), things go wrong.

"Glucose can't enter muscle cells as easily for use as fuel. So this excess circulating glucose that can't get inside your muscles indirectly triggers hunger hormones and you eat more, make more fat, and eventually gain weight," explains Liz Applegate, PhD, director of sports nutrition at University of California at Davis.

IN YOUR FAT CELLS: Your fat cells have internal sensors that help them keep track of how full they are. These sensors are similar to the one in your car's gas tank that triggers the fuel gauge to indicate that your tank is either full or empty. Vitamin D seems to help these sensors work properly. It's almost like a regular tune-up.

When D plugs into receptors on fat cells, it encourages the cells to secrete the hormone leptin. Leptin is an important hormone for you to understand. Many years ago, scientists thought it might be the solution to all body weight issues because it is a powerful hormone that seems to turn off hunger and turn up metabolism when it reaches the brain.

The problem, however, is that too much leptin might be worse than too little. When too much floods the brain on a regular basis, the brain stops responding to it, and this causes you to feel hungry all the time, even when you've just eaten.

Vitamin D seems to help normalize leptin and other hunger hormones, enabling fat cells to signal the brain to turn off the hunger sooner and longer.

IN YOUR BRAIN: When D plugs itself into receptors on brain cells, it stimulates the release of the mood-elevating chemical serotonin. "This improved mood and feeling of well-being helps people increase their level of activity and reduce their eating," explained Michael Holick, PhD, MD, from Boston University.

   In other words, you'll be more likely to lace up your sneakers and less likely to self-medicate with Blondies. The omega-3 fatty acids in the tuna and many other foods on this plan will also help to boost mood and emotional well-being.

Meal Replacement Shakes: They Go Right through You

IN YOUR MOUTH: Liquids pass through your mouth more quickly than Lady Gaga changes outfits. As a result, you will likely feel cheated when you come to the end of your can.

IN YOUR STOMACH: Unlike the taco, the meal replacement shake is both light and easy to digest. It moves quickly from the stomach to the intestine. Have you ever felt hungry within just an hour of drinking one of these? That's why. These beverages just don't stick around in the stomach long enough to provide lasting satisfaction. In contrast to most commercially available meal replacement beverages, you can make an incredibly filling smoothie at home. That's because you can load the smoothie up with low-calorie, high-fiber, and high-protein foods—all of which work to distend your stomach and trigger lasting fullness. *The 7-Day Slim Down* includes several smoothie recipes that do just that. These smoothies all contain some surprising yet satisfying ingredients, ranging from tofu to cauliflower to kefir to almond butter to cottage cheese. These ingredients have been artfully combined with fruit and other sweet-tasting foods to create a sweet-tasting drink that will fill you up fast and keep you satisfied for hours.

IN YOUR BLOODSTREAM: Think of the taco like a long-term, steady relationship. Think of the meal replacement shake as a one-night stand. It happens so quickly that you're not sure it even happened at all. Did you really drink it? Now you want another one just to be sure.

Because many of these beverages are formulated to be low glycemic, they do not generally cause large spikes in blood sugar. That's a good thing. They do, however, leave the intestine relatively quickly, so hunger hormones don't stay in check for very long.

Now not all meal replacement beverages are created equally. Some digest much more slowly than others because they have been supplemented with lots of fiber, protein, or both. If you have one that works for you, great. Go ahead and continue to use it. If not, opt for any of the smoothies on this plan. They are almost as convenient as commercially prepared meal replacement shakes, but they're much more satisfying for the reasons I've already mentioned.

IN YOUR FAT CELLS: If you manage to consume nothing other than your shake, you'll stay in a calorie deficit and be able to shed some fat. And that's why these beverages work so well for some dieters. They provide automatic portion control that takes the guesswork out of dieting.

But you've got to stick with it, and few people can. I don't think you need me to remind you of Oprah Winfrey's highly publicized regain after she lost weight with Opti-Fast. For many women, myself included, these meal replacement beverages just don't satisfy. They are great when you are in a rush, need something quick, and know you won't have time to think about the real food you never had the pleasure of eating. They are not so great when you are sitting at a dinner table with four companions, a lot of savory food, and your bottle of liquid calories. If you combine those liquid calories with solid ones, you'll end up plumping up your fat cells rather than slimming them down.

IN YOUR BRAIN: Depending on the makeup of your beverage, it might have little effect on your brain, or it might have a lot. If it's fortified with folic acid—an important B vitamin that some women lack—it could help to prevent depression. Beverages that are formulated to be low glycemic will help to stabilize mood better than those that are not.

These beverages have a much greater effect on the brain when you stop drinking them, though. I worked closely with world-renowned weight-loss expert Louis Aronne, MD, on his best-selling book, *The Skinny*. Dr. Aronne told me that he recommends a liquid diet for certain patients of his, especially those who are morbidly obese. This extremely low-calorie liquid diet is designed to help them shed pounds quickly and return them to good health as soon as possible. These patients drink shakes for months. They are highly motivated because they know what they are looking at: If they don't lose weight with the shakes, their next stop is surgery. So they generally do great on the liquid diet.

But eventually they reach their goals and it's time to bring solid food back into the picture. Dr. Aronne told me that he must coach people through this transition because it's one that is fraught with the potential to backslide. Because the patients have had nothing but liquids for so long, chemicals in their brains, called endocan-nabinoids, are especially sensitive. These chemicals, responsible for making food such a pleasurable experience, rise when we eat. When people break a liquid fast, Dr. Aronne tells me, these chemicals rise dramatically at the first taste of solid food. Food suddenly tastes better than it has ever tasted before because these chemicals are flooding the brain with pleasure. Dr. Aronne prescribes the most boring meal on the planet to his patients who break their liquid fast. It's skinless chicken breast. Yet, without fail, the patients tell him that the skinless chicken breast was the best chicken they've had in their entire lives. It's really no different than any other chicken breast they've ever eaten, but the endocannabinoids are so high in their brains that even packing peanuts would taste divine.

Ice Cream and Chips: Holy Overeating!

IN YOUR MOUTH: Your taste buds communicate with your brain, giving it information about the food's flavor and texture. Based on this information, your brain will either turn up or turn down your pleasure response. Certain flavors—bitter, spicy, and sour—will cause your brain to turn down the pleasure response relatively quickly, so you lose interest in eating. Other flavors, such as the yummy sweet-and-salty combination of the ice cream and chips, cause the pleasure response to stay elevated for a much longer time. This may be yet another leftover evolutionary trait, as bitter- and sour-tasting foods tended to contain harmful substances and sweet-tasting foods tended to contain the energy needed to sustain life—especially during drought, famine, and hard times.

But this evolutionary response is one reason it's so hard to stop eating crunchy, salty foods like chips and creamy, sweet foods like ice cream. Even when your stomach feels uncomfortably full, your brain is still broadcasting pleasure, so you keep telling yourself, "Okay, just one more bite." When you combine sweet with salty, you put your brain in an ice cream–induced nirvana state for quite a while, spooning the stuff into your mouth as you stand in front of the sink and stare blankly into space.

IN YOUR STOMACH: Ice cream and chips pack a lot of calories into a small space. They are light foods, too. By that, I mean they are light in weight, not in calories. As a result, it takes a lot more of both foods to weigh down your stomach and trigger a sensation of fullness than it takes bites of taco.

IN YOUR BLOODSTREAM: Ice cream and chips move through your intestine and into your bloodstream faster than Michael Phelps can swim the length of a kiddie pool. Once all of that sugar from the ice cream makes its way through your intestinal wall and into your bloodstream, glucose levels start to rise quickly. The human body tries very hard to keep blood glucose levels steady, so as levels rise, the pancreas secretes gobs of the hormone insulin.

As a result, way more insulin than is needed floods the bloodstream. Blood sugar levels drop quickly, dipping to levels that are below normal. Blood sugar levels are closely tied to hunger levels.

As blood sugar drops, hunger sets in. This is why you can feel hungry not very long after eating a lot more ice cream than you know you should have eaten—and, as I can tell you from experience, it's pretty frustrating!

IN YOUR FAT CELLS: As I mentioned earlier, the ice cream is going to spike insulin, which is going to escort all of that excess sugar and fat to any cell it can find—including your fat cells. This is why some foods are literally more fattening than others. A 500-calorie meal that causes an insulin surge (like ice cream) is far more likely to end up housed in your fat cells than a 500-calorie meal that causes a slow, even rise in insulin (like a tuna taco).

IN YOUR BRAIN: The rebound hunger caused by the sugar in the ice cream will also cause rebound depression and fatigue in your brain. You'll feel elated for a short time as the sugar works to boost mood. Then your mood will plummet and you will find yourself feeling grumpy, sad, and fatigued.

How to Reduce Hunger Even More

THE TUNA TACO is just one of dozens of options that will help you fill up on fewer calories. This plan maximizes your consumption of fiber, protein, vitamin D, and many other filling nutrients, minimizing the hunger and cravings that may have derailed your diet efforts in the past. These foods work together to weigh down your stomach—triggering those stretch receptors to send fullness signals to your brain. They trigger the release of fullness hormones in your intestine. They make your cells more sensitive to insulin. They keep blood sugar steady. They boost mood and they help you stick with the plan long term.

Here are additional strategies you can use to boost satisfaction and keep hunger in check.

➜ **Get plenty of sleep.** Lack of sleep plays havoc with a number of hormones that can increase your hunger. When you don't get enough sleep, levels of the hunger hormone ghrelin rise as levels of the satiety hormone leptin fall. This causes your brain to turn up your sensations of hunger and your cravings for sweet, fatty foods (like donuts and brownies). The drop in leptin also slows your metabolism, so your body burns fewer calories at rest. It also can lead to insulin resistance, causing more blood sugar to get stored in your fat cells. Lack of sleep also causes the stress hormone cortisol to rise, triggering much of that fat to go to your tummy.

A Kaiser Permanente study found that people trying to lose at least 10 pounds were more likely to reach that goal if they had lower stress levels and slept more than 6 hours a night. "This study suggests that when people are trying to lose weight, they should try to get the right amount of sleep and reduce their stress," said lead author Charles Elder, MD, MPH, an investigator with the Kaiser Permanente Center for Health Research in Portland, Oregon; he also leads Integrative Medicine at Kaiser Permanente Northwest. "Some people may just need to cut back on their schedules and get to bed earlier. Others may find that exercise can reduce stress and help them sleep. For some people, mind/body techniques such as meditation also might be helpful."

Another study done at Walter Reed Army Medical Center in Washington, DC, found that people who slept fewer than 6 hours at night tended to

CHEW ON THIS

At any given time, you only have about 40 calories' worth of glucose in your blood. This is only enough energy to keep you alive for a few minutes, which is why you feel so hungry when blood glucose levels drop below normal. It's also why you feel dizzy and can't concentrate when you go on a starvation diet. Your blood glucose is low most of the time.

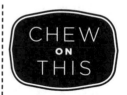

weigh more than people who slept more—even though these sleep skimpers power walked an extra 1.5 miles a day. And a Harvard study of 68,000 women determined that women who got just 5 hours of sleep at night were 32 percent more likely to gain 33 pounds over 16 years than women who got 7 hours of shut-eye or more.

I could go on and on here, citing study after study after study. Sleep is important, not just for your diet, but for your overall health. We all need more of it.

➡ **Get stress under control.** Like lack of sleep, stress can also lead to hunger, as the Kaiser Permanente study previously mentioned shows. In addition to increasing hunger and cravings, stress raises levels of cortisol, a hormone that directs the body to store fat in your abdomen. Regular exercise can help get stress under control, which is one reason exercise is so important in any weight-loss regimen. Meditation and relaxation exercises help, too. In one study done at the University of California, a 4-month mindfulness meditation program was able to curb weight gain in 47 women, whereas stressed women who did not meditate continued to gain weight.

➡ **Use vinegar to flavor salads and other foods.** Acetic acid is the ingredient that gives vinegar its sour taste. It also slows the rate of stomach emptying, so your food takes longer to break down into the very small particles that can travel through your intestinal wall and into your bloodstream. When consumed with food, vinegar has been shown to reduce the glycemic response to what you eat by a whopping 50 to 55 percent. As a result, it seems to reduce appetite. In one study, participants who consumed a diluted vinegar drink ate 12 percent less for the rest of the day (the equivalent of roughly 200 calories). And 2 daily tablespoons of red raspberry vinegar doubled weight loss over 2 weeks.

➡ **Spice up with cinnamon.** Studies suggest that cinnamon may have a stabilizing effect on blood sugar levels, which could curtail appetite. I like to sprinkle it on everything from plain yogurt to fruit.

➡ **Eat mindfully.** There's a lag between the time your stomach fills with food and the time it takes for the "full" signal to reach your brain and switch off your sensation of hunger. The more quickly you eat, the more likely you will finish everything on your plate and still feel hungry. The more slowly you eat, the more likely you will feel full and satisfied once you've finished your portion. You'll also feel more satisfied if you actually notice that you are eating. Try to notice the first bite, a few bites in the middle, and the very last bite.

Now you know how the 7-Day Slim Down turns up fat burning and dials down hunger. There's just one more piece of the successful weight loss puzzle: motivation. Without it you're nowhere. In the next chapter you'll learn how the foods you'll be eating will help you stay on track and become a part of your lean, healthy lifestyle for good.

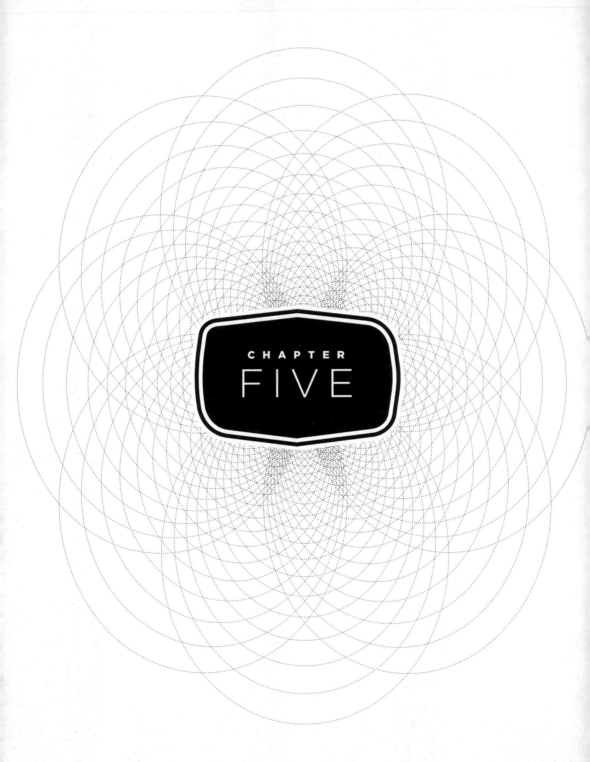

CHAPTER
FIVE

How You'll Stay Motivated

I'm going to tell you something that most diet authors won't. It's this: You can lose weight on practically any diet. It doesn't matter if it's low carb or low fat or low ice cream. It doesn't matter if the diet features grapefruit, acai berries, or peanut butter. It doesn't matter if the diet requires you to consume only raw foods, only liquid foods, or only vegetarian foods.

You can lose weight on any of them, and in fact, you probably have in the past. If you only want to lose weight, it truly doesn't matter what diet you try. Any of them can work for you—for a while, anyway. Yet, depending on how much weight you want to lose, it can take weeks, months, and sometimes even years to finally get the body you want. And then you need to follow a version of that plan for life in order to prevent the pounds from creeping back on. The problem with most diets, however, is this: They are not sustainable long-term.

Can you eat raw for life? Can you avoid bread and pasta for life? Can you periodically fast or cleanse or go liquid for life?

I can't, and I'm not ashamed to admit it.

Indeed, perhaps one of the most important characteristics of a winning diet is this: It's something you can follow without feeling the urge to cheat. Think about it. How many diets have you stuck to religiously—without cheating, without backsliding, without relapsing, and without eventually regaining? I'm guessing none of them. Otherwise, you wouldn't be reading this book.

But don't blame yourself for that. Blame the diets.

If you've "failed" at diets in the past, it's really not your fault. You are not a bad dieter. You are not weak or lazy. The diets you've tried in the past did not prepare you mentally and physically to follow them long term.

The 7-Day Slim Down is different. It's designed to help you stay motivated and follow the plan for as long as you need or want to. I've made sure to include a variety of foods and menus so you will never feel deprived of the foods you love. I've even built cheating strategies into the plan, to help you feel confident no matter where you find yourself: at restaurants, on vacation, out with your girl-friends, or at Thanksgiving with your food-obsessed family.

Dieting—even with a well-designed diet like this one—isn't easy. If sticking to a diet were easy, more than 60 percent of people in the United States wouldn't be overweight. It's hard to change your lifestyle. It takes courage, dedication, an ability to problem solve, and more. That's why, in the following pages, I'll show you how the 7-Day Slim Down ensures success by fueling you with crucial nutrients to boost your willpower—as well as additional strategies, tips, and tricks you can use to tackle any dieting dilemma and still stay on track!

The Ingredients of Willpower

SO WHAT HELPS you stick to one diet and not to another? It all comes down to a cost benefit analysis. As long as the benefits far outweigh the costs, you will have an easier time sticking to the diet. If the costs start to outweigh the benefits, however, your willpower will start to erode.

Many diets try to hide their costs. I'm not going to do that. You're smart, savvy, and don't need to be tricked. Let's be honest, there are costs to sticking to any diet, including this one. You will have to get used to eating new foods and making unfamiliar meals. It might take a little longer to shop for groceries and prepare meals. Fortunately, these are relatively minor costs and will become virtually nonexistent the longer you stick to the plan.

I've attempted to minimize any feelings of deprivation on this plan by allowing you to eat a serving of any food—no matter how junky—once a day. Still, you will probably be eating less of something. There's no sugar-coating this. Perhaps your portions will be smaller

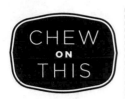
*When research-
ers at the
Pennington
Biomedical
Research Center
at Louisiana
State University
compared
four different
diets, they found
that it was
adherence—
how well partici-
pants followed
any given diet—
that predicted
success. If
participants
followed the diet
as prescribed,
they lost the
most weight over
6 months.*

than what you are used to. Maybe you will be eating less dessert than you'd like or have fewer glasses of wine. Over time, though, your body will adjust to this new way of eating—and you'll start to enjoy the way you look and feel.

Finally, I would be lying if I told you that you would never feel hungry again. You likely will, especially at the very beginning of the program. But the meal plans in this book ensure that you'll choose from satisfying foods that fill you up and curb hunger as much as possible.

These costs exist, and it's important to acknowledge them. But the good news is that the benefits of this plan far outweigh the costs. In addition to sculpting a gorgeously slim shape and seeing results almost immediately, you'll boost your mood and increase your energy levels—two key ingredients to staying motivated.

How You'll Stay Happy

IF YOU'RE ANYTHING like me, then the long, cold, dark days of winter can suck the willpower out of you like a self-absorbed talkaholic sucks the energy out of a room. That's probably due, in part, to the winter blues.

Reduced sunlight disrupts your body's natural circadian clock—also known as your sleep-wake clock. Changes in sunlight seem to disrupt two important hormones: melatonin and serotonin. Melatonin is a hormone that your brain releases

ARE YOU
SAD?

If you suffer from five or more of the following during the winter,
you might have full-blown Seasonal Affective Disorder.
If fewer than five are true, you might still have a milder form:

○ DEPRESSION

○ LOSS OF INTEREST IN
ACTIVITIES

○ WEIGHT FLUCTUATIONS

○ INSOMNIA OR HYPERSOMNIA

○ POOR CONCENTRATION

○ FATIGUE

○ REPETITIVE AGITATED MOVE-
MENTS, SUCH AS PACING OR
WRINGING OF THE HANDS

○ FEELINGS OF WORTHLESS-
NESS, GUILT, OR SHAME

○ SUICIDAL THOUGHTS

at night to induce sleep; serotonin is a nervous system chemical that affects mood, appetite, and sleep. When levels of both are too low, it can lead to a kind of depression called Seasonal Affective Disorder (SAD).

This depression usually strikes during the winter, when the days are short and light is scarce. It occurs in women more than in men and seems to be influenced by body temperature, genetics, and hormones. It starts in late autumn and can lead to increased appetite and cravings—especially for carbs. This obviously makes it difficult to stick to a diet! It also causes increased sleepiness and low energy, both of which make it hard to exercise consistently. And it often causes poor concentration, especially in the afternoon.

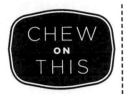

*Women are
more likely to
get SAD than
men. It's also
more common
in people who
live far from
the equator,
probably due
to decreased
sunlight.*

SAD is a medical disorder that affects roughly 6 percent of the population. (That sounds like a small percentage, but consider that it only includes people with issues severe enough to have required a doctor's care.) It's thought that roughly 20 percent of women—about one in every five women—have a milder form of SAD. And physicians now believe that most people experience some seasonal variations in mood and energy levels.

Whether you have a mild or a severe form of SAD, there are several ways that the 7-Day Slim Down can help.

YOU'LL BOOST MOOD WITH EVEN MORE D. This program features two different menu plans—one for the summer, when sunlight is more plentiful, and another for the winter, when the days are short. Due to the lack of sunlight, you need more D during the winter months. Some experts theorize that a drop in D during the winter may be what's actually behind SAD in the first place. Consider that:

➜ Your brain is full of vitamin D receptors.
➜ Low levels of D have been linked with higher levels of cytokines. Cytokines are proteins that increase inflammation and have been shown to be a possible risk factor for depression.
➜ Studies have found that low levels of vitamin D are associated with higher levels of depression. For instance, Italian women with lower blood levels of vitamin D had twice the risk of developing depression as women with higher levels.

➜ Supplemental D has been shown to relieve symptoms of depression, and the relief seems to come quickly, in as few as 5 days.

YOU'LL CONSUME PLENTY OF FISH. This plan is loaded with fatty fish, a rich source of D and omega-3 fatty acids. Omega-3s are an important type of fat that has been shown to play a big role in brain health. These fats are highly concentrated in the brain and play a role in memory, mental performance, and mood. People who are deficient in omega-3 fatty acids tend to suffer from fatigue, muddled thinking, mood swings, and depression. Over the past 20 years, our consumption of omega-3 fatty acids has dropped and rates of depression have risen.

YOU'LL GET THE RIGHT AMOUNT OF CALCIUM. Like D, calcium is an important mood booster as well as a sleep enabler.

MORE MOOD-BOOSTING STRATEGIES

SNACK SMART. Instead of sweet desserts, make any of the following natural mood boosters part of your snacking repertoire: dates, bananas, or papayas. They all contain the right balance of amino acids to boost serotonin levels in the brain without leading to a rebound drop.

GET UP AND OUT. Make it a habit to go for a brief walk (or jog) outdoors first thing in the morning, for up to 30 minutes, if possible. Not only will this kick off your day with an extra boost of sunlight (depending on the weather), you'll also find that the fresh air will invigorate your senses and the exercise will go a long way toward keeping your energy levels high all day.

CONSIDER LIGHT THERAPY. Light therapy involves using a special box that mimics outdoor sunlight, helping to trick your brain into operating as if it were still summer. I keep one on my desk and turn it on in the morning so I can dose myself with light for 30 minutes to an hour while I work.

These lights are available from many online retailers and sometimes can be purchased from health professionals too. If you decide to get one, make sure the box you purchase provides 10,000 lux. Work with your doctor to find the best dosage for you, but 30 minutes each morning is the most typical recommendation. Light therapy should start to lift depression in a few weeks to a month, but you will notice some effects right away. For instance you will start to feel more energetic almost as soon as you turn on the box.

Note: Do not use light therapy if you are taking medications that increase your sensitivity to sunlight or if you have bipolar disorder. Also, consult an eye doctor before starting treatment, as the light can affect your eyes.

LET THE LIGHT IN. Do whatever you can to safely maximize sunlight in your daily life. Keep the blinds open during the winter. Trim trees and bushes around the outside of your house to avoid too much shade. Sit closer to windows in restaurants during the day. Take breaks at work to step outside—even just for a few minutes—if it's sunny out.

TALK TO YOUR DOCTOR. If you feel you suffer from a more severe case of SAD, you might benefit from an antidepressant during the winter months. Know that some antidepressants cause weight gain. According to Manhattan diet doctor Louis Aronne, MD, this problem can be solved by working with your doctor and adjusting your medications. For instance, Dr. Aronne says Wellbutrin (bupropion) tends to induce weight loss, whereas many other antidepressants have the opposite effect. Wellbutrin XL is an extended release medication that has been shown to prevent SAD.

It's important to start treatment before SAD symptoms set in. For instance, you might need to start treatment as early as August each year.

How You'll Stay Energized

The lack of sunlight in the winter months doesn't just affect your mood; it can also bring on some serious fatigue. I don't know about you, but when it gets dark by 4 p.m., I'm a lot more likely to want to relax on the couch in my favorite fleece PJs than I am to hit the gym or even go for a short walk.

This kind of winter fatigue can also bring on massive cravings. Have you ever tried to eat through your fatigue? If you have, then you know what I'm talking about. It all might start innocently enough with something like baby carrots. Then come the graham crackers. And then the nuts. And then the cheese, and then those big, chewy chocolate chip cookies that you really wanted all along.

By normalizing levels of vitamin D, you'll be able to combat winter fatigue and curb these cravings. The extra D you'll be consuming during the winter months will help boost energy in the following ways:

➤ There are D receptors on your muscles, so getting enough D helps you to succeed in your exercise efforts. Your results will serve as a reward to keep you going.

➤ People who are deficient in D tend to have unexplained aches and pains in their joints and muscles. D helps you feel good so you are more likely to exercise and less likely to lie around and think about food.

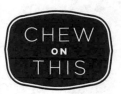

CHEW
ON
THIS

D can also help with more serious cases of fatigue that might be caused by medical issues, such as chronic fatigue syndrome (CFS). When researchers in London tested D levels in 221 women with chronic fatigue syndrome, the women with CFS were all low in D, compared to another group of women without CFS who weren't low in D.

➜ A study by Atascadero State Hospital in Atascadero, California, found that athletic performance improved when D levels were brought up to optimal levels.

➜ The American Society of Anesthesiologists released a report in October of 2007 that found one in four patients with chronic pain issues were deficient in D. Their study also found that those with lower levels of vitamin D required higher doses of morphine over a longer period of time.

MORE ENERGY-BOOSTING STRATEGIES

LOWER YOUR EXPECTATIONS. It's easy to confuse comfort with fatigue. In other words, you may think you're "way too tired to work out," when really, you're just more comfortable inside a cozy, warm house. To keep your excuse-generating self in check, never allow yourself to give in to the "too tired" excuse completely. Rather than completely blowing off a workout, tell yourself, "Okay, I'll just do 5 minutes instead of 30," or "I'll go to the gym, but if I'm still too tired after 5 minutes on the elliptical, then I'm done." Often, 99 percent of the battle is just getting out of the house. If you set simple, easy expectations, you'll be more likely to lace up your sneakers and get going. Chances are, once you start moving, you won't stop after just 5 minutes.

GET FRESH AIR. Even just standing outdoors (whether it's sunny or not) can wake you up enough to make you feel more energetic. Whenever you are tempted to self-medicate your fatigue with food, tell yourself, "No, I'll just step outside for a minute." Once you're out there, take a few deep breaths. Chances are, that will be all you need to stimulate your system and boost your energy levels.

HYDRATE. Whether it's heat or air conditioning, indoor ventilation systems can be drying, and dehydration can lead to tiredness and the

cravings that come with it. Sip water with lemon, or drink warm herbal tea throughout the day to stay hydrated and fend off fatigue.

How You'll Stay Motivated

The 7-Day Slim Down helps you stay motivated in part by feeding your body with the ingredients it needs to stay in a good mood and energized. It also makes it easy to enjoy all of the benefits of this program—namely, lasting weight loss—by allowing you to customize and configure the diet plan to truly fit your needs. As a result, you'll feel confident about your ability to succeed and stick to the plan no matter what the situation.

RAPID RESULTS. By helping you fill up on fewer calories, the 7-Day Slim Down will go a long, long way toward helping you stay on track. By filling your plate with the world's most satisfying foods, you'll be better able to put down your fork and push away from the table long before you've overeaten. As a result, you'll enjoy watching the numbers on the scale drop more quickly than ever.

A FEELING OF CONTROL. Rather than forcing you to follow a set menu day after day, I worked hard to give you options and show you how to make substitutions. I know there will be times when you just don't want to eat another piece of fish, for instance. As a result, I've provided advice on how to swap the fish for whatever source of protein you are in the mood for, whether it's chicken, beef, or something else.

COMFORT FOODS WHEN YOU NEED THEM MOST. The last thing I want to eat during the dark, cold winter months is a salad or a smoothie.

Yet the vast majority of diets seem to expect people to be able to eat light foods like this no matter what time of year it is. This plan offers specific food strategies for both winter and summer, understanding that your tastes will change with the seasons. The winter plan is chock-full of options that will satisfy your winter yearnings for comfort and warmth. You'll find soups, stews, and more. And the summer plan offers lighter, more refreshing choices.

AN EXERCISE PLAN YOU CAN LIVE WITH. Like the menu plans, the exercise plan is full of options that you can customize to fit your lifestyle. You'll find muscle-firming options you can do at home or at the gym. Couple that with some cardio—especially cardio done outdoors in sunlight—and you'll create a winning plan you can follow for life.

MORE SUPER-MOTIVATING STRATEGIES

DO: TALK TO YOUR HOUSEHOLD. Whether you live with kids or roommates, it's important to get everyone on the same page regarding the food you're cooking and eating. You may be making some significant changes to the contents of the fridge and pantry. Remind your household that this diet isn't just for you to lose weight. It's for everyone to eat healthier, too. Expect to hear some gripes and grumbles for a week or two. But eventually, everyone will see that you mean business—and they'll probably start to enjoy the delicious meals along with you (even if they don't admit it!).

DO: RALLY YOUR SUPPORT TEAM. The more support you have, the better. You might ask your spouse to take a walk with you each night after dinner, for instance. Or perhaps you can find co-workers who are also looking to lose weight, and you can eat lunch together. Surround yourself with upbeat, like-minded people, and don't be afraid to let someone know if they're being pushy with food or just negative. To anyone who doesn't actively support you, try saying this: "I really need your help to make sure I succeed on this diet. Are you willing to help me do this?"

DO: CREATE A MEAL-ENDING RITUAL. I like to end my meals with a cup of hot tea. It takes a while to sip the tea, which mentally gives me time to adjust to the fact that the meal is over. Maybe you take a walk after dinner each night. Maybe you clean the kitchen. Do whatever works for you to help you shift out of eating mode.

DO: WALK OFF CRAVINGS. Walking for 15 minutes has been shown to decrease cravings among smokers. Other research found that 2 weeks of regular exercise induced changes in the brain that suppressed cravings. Whenever you feel the urge to snack but you're not truly hungry, take a lap or two around the block and clear your head.

DO: EAT BEFORE YOU ARE TRULY HUNGRY. As ghrelin levels go up, willpower goes down. Research shows that dieters tend to make fattening food choices when they are hungry. That's when they reach for high-calorie, high-fat foods. The less hungry you feel just before a meal, the more likely you are to make appropriate food choices. (This is the same rationale behind why you're not supposed to grocery shop when you're hungry.) As you are losing weight, it's also a good idea to shift your meals, especially dinner, a bit earlier. This allows you to eat before you are starving, so you are better able to stay in control. You also might find that this helps to improve your sleep, as you will have fully digested dinner before going to bed.

DO: SHIFT FROM GUILT TO TRIUMPH. Telling yourself things like "this is so fattening" will only serve to reduce your willpower even more. Instead, shift from negative to positive and tell yourself how good it felt to slip into that cute cocktail dress without a struggle!

DO: THINK LONG-TERM. Weight loss is usually hardest in the beginning. That's when you are still getting used to change. To help yourself overcome the stress of change, try this little trick that I learned from Manhattan psychotherapist Jonathan Alpert, author of the book *Be Fearless*. Create a pay-off list. On it, write all of the reasons you've decided to lose weight. Whether it's fitting into your skinny jeans, losing baby weight, having a better sex life, or improving your overall health—or all of the above! Carry your list with you and look at it whenever you are tempted to call it quits. Your list will remind you of why you have chosen to do this and it will help you look beyond the short-term stress you're facing.

DO: EAT BEFORE EXERCISE. Is there a particular junk food that tends to unravel your sense of control? Try eating it just before a very intense exercise session. Doing so might cause you to lose your taste for it. When Dutch researchers asked 58 participants to consume different flavored drinks just before a 30-minute run, the participants developed an aversion to the flavor of the drink. This is similar to how you might feel about the last food you ate before you got sick with the stomach flu. You associate the flavor of the food with discomfort, and as a result, you stop liking it.

DO: KEEP A FOOD DIARY. University of Pittsburgh researchers have found that dieters who consistently jot down what they eat lose weight more quickly than dieters who do not. And research from the same school found that keeping a food diary helped dieters follow their diets more religiously without backsliding or cheating, even after a full year.

Food diaries work because they make you more conscious of all of your closet nibbling. Your diary can also help you pinpoint certain foods that might trigger rebound hunger or cravings. For instance, some research shows that cheese can produce chemical reactions in the brains of some people that block the brain's satiety response—leaving them feeling hungrier and having more cravings for a full 48 hours.

If you decide to keep a food diary, make sure that it can travel with you wherever you eat. Diet-tracker apps are a great idea since they're right on your phone. If it's relevant, jot down notes about your mood (happy, relaxed, stressed, angry) and the type of day you are having (boring, busy, hard, easy). At the end of each week, review your diary and note what seems to be making you stay on track, or make adjustments based on your needs.

DO: EAT TEMPTING FOODS WITH YOUR NONDOMINANT HAND. This will slow down your pace of eating and make you more aware of every bite, giving you more chances to stop before it's too late. Another common strategy that works: using chopsticks!

DO: PUT A MIRROR IN YOUR DINING ROOM. One study found that eating in front of mirrors slashed the amount people ate by nearly one-third. The mirror technique might work by making you accountable to your own goals (not to mention your own reflection!).

DO: THINK POSITIVE. Prepare an affirmation that you will repeat to yourself whenever you feel tempted to eat more than your designated portion. It might be as simple as, "I'm full. I don't need to eat more," or it might be more symbolic, like, "I am strong. I can resist this and make a better choice."

DO: USE SMALLER PLATES. Research shows that we feel more satisfied when food fills up the space on our plates. When you use regular dinner plates, your portions look small. The same is true for drinking glasses and bowls. Switch to smaller appetizer or dessert plates and bowls and you will have a much easier time feeling satisfied.

DO: DISTRACT YOURSELF. When you feel the urge to eat between meals or to help yourself to seconds, distract yourself with a quick activity. Most urges will pass within about 20 minutes. Take care of a few household chores. Call a friend. Do something that takes your mind off eating and food. Chances are, once some times goes by, you'll completely forget that you wanted to eat in the first place.

DO: HIDE TEMPTING FOODS. Just seeing or smelling food can trigger a response in your brain that makes you feel hungry, even when you've just eaten. Override this response by plating your meal and then putting the rest away—out of sight. Don't keep serving bowls on the table. If the rest of your family tends to eat seconds, then eat with your family in the dining room, but keep the serving bowls in the kitchen. And request that someone else help with cleanup duty—especially with leftovers. (Perhaps you cooked, so it's a fair trade, or you can handle another household chore.) Similarly, keep overly tempting snack foods, such as chocolate and wine, out of sight. When you want to indulge, pour yourself a glass or break off a serving. Then immediately put the rest away where you can't see it.

DO: EAT YOUR MOST TEMPTING FOOD AT THE SAME TIME EVERY DAY. Research shows that eating the same flavor day after day tends to cause our brains to tire of that flavor, turning down the pleasure response to that food. So if you tend to lose control with a specific food, like chocolate, eating it every day at the same time may help you to gain more control over your cravings. The first day will be the hardest, so take extra precautions. Measure out the correct portion and pack only that amount as your snack or meal. Then, eat it some- where relaxing and possibly with another person present—someone you trust to stop you from searching for more! It's also important to eat tempting indulgence foods after a meal. That way, the other food in your GI tract will slow the absorption of sugar into your bloodstream, preventing the highs and lows that can lead to cravings and bingeing. Do this every day for a week and you'll start to feel increased self-control.

DO: REMEMBER DON'T ATTEMPT TO HATE YOURSELF THIN. In a study done in Portugal, 239 overweight or obese women who completed a body image program lost more weight than those who didn't. The body image program encouraged the women to focus on weight loss not as a way to become sexier or more beautiful or likeable, but rather as a way to become stronger and healthier. The women learned to stop calling themselves things like "fat cow" (how awful!) and stopped using other negative words, too.

Many women also talk down to themselves . How many times have I heard, "I should have," or "I have to," when talking about dieting or eating healthfully? This kind of language implies a loss of control, and when you use it—even silently in your head—it erodes your motivation, making you feel as if the diet controls you rather than the other way around.

It's much more motivating to use phrases like, "I want to," "I choose to," and "I've decided to." Such phrases put you in charge. When you use them ("I've decided to have a banana-strawberry shake"), you feel in control, and you are more likely to execute your dieting choices over the long term. When researchers from the Duke University Diet and Fitness Center kept tabs on 252 of their patients after they were discharged from the treatment center, they discovered that positive self-talk (telling yourself I can do this, I want to do this, I will do this, I deserve to do this) was one of the top three strategies the most successful dieters used to lose weight and keep it off. (By the way, planning meals and keeping a food diary were the other top strategies.)

It's my hope that you are feeling confident about the food plan you're about to embark on. I've provided you with the scientific support and explanations you need to feel confident that this plan works—and works quickly. There's just one more bit of knowledge to absorb. In Chapter 6, you'll learn about the plan's star foods and how they work together to melt fat, reduce hunger, and help you feel fantastic.

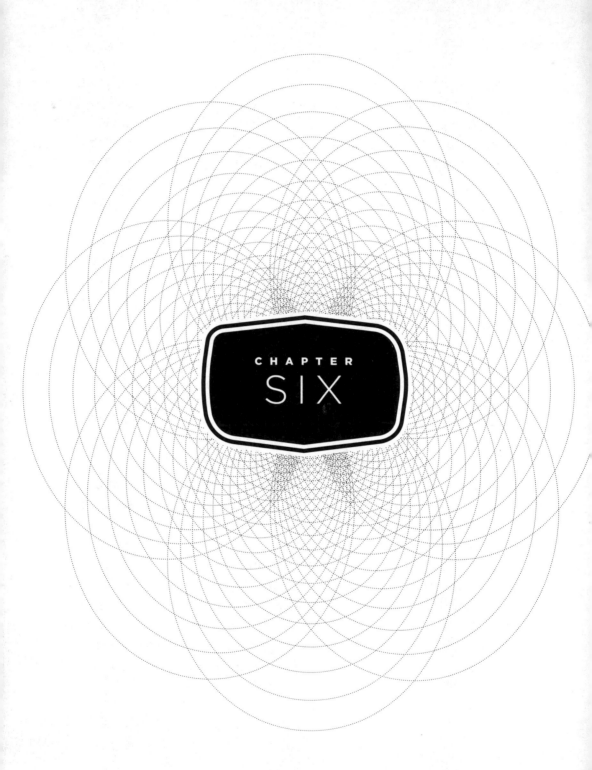

CHAPTER

SIX

The Top
ght
ming
ods

Eau Claire Distillery
distillery

好喝的了，舒服了

Until very recently, you couldn't find much vitamin D in the foods you consumed on a regular basis. Most of the natural sources of D—such as liver, kidney, and other organ meats—are foods that few people consume on a regular basis. And many other foods only house scant amounts of D. As a result, it was nearly impossible to consume all the D you needed through diet alone. You needed the sun and supplements just to keep your D levels up to the minimum requirements.

In recent years, thankfully, this has all changed for the better. As the importance of D has emerged, more and more fortified products have been hitting the market. D is now found in much more than just the milk you drink. It's in some OJs, breads, cereals, and even SpaghettiOs. At the same time, agricultural experts have found ways to add huge doses of D to certain types of foods—especially eggs and mushrooms. By feeding hens a special diet, they've been able to, for example, create eggs with double the usual amount of D. And by harvesting mushrooms in sunlight rather than darkness, they've been able to actually quintuple their D content.

It's easier and easier to meet your D requirements through diet. This is a good thing, too, because food provides powerful weight-loss benefits that supplements cannot. Unlike supplements, foods are housed in a complete package where several nutrients work synergistically to affect hunger, metabolism, mood, and much more. Consume the right combination of nutrients and you can more easily melt fat. Consume the wrong combination and you are faced with intense hunger, cravings, and a sluggish metabolism.

The decision is pretty clear to me. And that is: I'd rather eat my way to a smaller waistline.

While it's becoming more possible to eat large quantities of D, it's not quite a nutritionally sound plan. To meet your D requirement through food alone, you would have to consume a lot of one food in particular: salmon. You might be able to eat and enjoy salmon at the start of a diet, but every day for the rest of your life? I doubt it. And that's precisely why this food plan recommends that you take a supplement. A daily D supplement of 1,000 to 2,000 IU during the winter months reduces your need to stay 100 percent true to the plan and allows you to occasionally have lower D days in your diet.

All of that said, you will see eight foods over and over again on the menus in this book. They are all powerful slimming packages that contain several nutrients that work together to boost metabolism and reduce hunger. Let's take a closer look at how these nutrients work.

FISH

In a study done many years ago in Australia, overweight patients who ate fish daily as part of a weight-loss regimen lost more weight than others who were dieting but not consuming fish. Fish houses a trifecta of slimming nutrients.

VITAMIN D: Many types of fish are among the foods richest in D, with some varieties providing nearly 1,000 IU of D per serving.

PROTEIN: Fish is high in protein, which helps to satisfy and suppress appetite. Protein also helps to balance blood sugar levels and may help turn up your metabolism after meals.

OMEGA-3 FATTY ACIDS: Fatty fish are one of the few food sources of this ultraimportant fat (nuts and flaxseeds are the other sources). Omega-3 fatty acids are known as essential fats because our bodies can't make them. Various studies show that many people are not getting enough, which can lead to an array of health problems. Studies show that high doses of this fat can speed metabolism

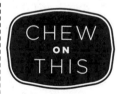

CHEW
ON
THIS

Vitamin D is relatively stable in food—storage and cooking have little effect on it, even when it's heated to boiling temperatures of 212°F. This means you'll get all the nutritional benefits of these fat-blasting foods no matter how you prepare them!

by as much as 400 calories a day. Omega-3s have been shown to prevent dangerous blood clots, improve blood cholesterol levels, and help manage chronic diseases such as psoriasis, migraine headaches, and arthritis. These fats might help to lift depression, too.

Certain types of fish—especially small, bony fish like anchovies—are also a rich source of calcium, a slimmer I've already told you about.

These nutrients and more make fish and shellfish two of your most potent fat-melting allies. People who consume fish-rich diets have healthier insulin and blood sugar levels than people who consume diets low in fish. In one study done in Iceland, people who consumed fish three times a week had more beneficial insulin levels during weight loss than dieters who didn't consume fish. As I've mentioned, insulin levels are important. When insulin levels are stable, hunger is low and fat burning is high.

A diet high in fish might also help to block the formation of new fat cells as well as trigger the body to waste calories as heat. The mood-boosting effect of omega-3 fatty acids alone can go a long way toward keeping a lid on cravings. Fish and shellfish are low-calorie foods. Lobster adds only 83 calories per 3 ounces and shrimp just 60 calories per 12 large shrimp. Even fatty fish like salmon is relatively low in calories when you compare it to steak and other types of meat. This allows you to consume larger portions, which makes you feel more satisfied.

Finally, some types of fish and shellfish—especially shrimp, crab, and oysters—slow eating because you must remove them from the shell. This allows more time for the fullness signal to reach the brain.

PICK FATTY FISH, NOT LEAN FISH: Not all fish are created equal. As I've mentioned, vitamin D is a fat-soluble vitamin. That means it prefers to hang out in fat. Vitamin D is concentrated in the fatty parts of fish. It's for this reason that fatty fish contain more D than leaner varieties do. Lean varieties of fish like flounder contain about 118 IU per 3-ounce serving. Fatty fish like salmon offer four times that amount. Fatty fish are also a richer source of omega-3 fatty acids.

How much D a fish contains depends on other factors as well, ranging from the natural diet of the fish to where the fish was harvested. The chart that follows will give you a rough idea of how much D certain varieties of fish contain. For a more extensive list of fish that are high in D, see the Appendix.

VARIETY OF FISH (3.5-OUNCE SERVING)	IU OF D
WILD SALMON	988
AHI TUNA	404
FARMED TROUT	388
BLUEFISH	280
FARMED SALMON	240
SOLE	56

PICK WILD SALMON, NOT FARM-RAISED: A Boston University study found that farmed salmon only contained 25 percent of the D that its wild cousins had. Wild salmon get D from eating D-rich plankton and have approximately 800 to 1,000 IU of vitamin D in 3.5 ounces. Farmed salmon, which eat feed pellets low in D, have only 10 to 25 percent of this amount.

LEARN EASY WAYS TO MAKE FISH. For instance, it doesn't get any easier than grilled wild salmon. Take 3.5 ounces of it, lightly brush the fish with olive oil, then sprinkle it with salt and pepper. Grill the fish, skin side down, for about 5 minutes, flip and grill until the fish flakes when prodded with a fork—just 3 to 5 minutes more. Or you can bake or broil it. Finally, for tender fish, consider boiling it in vegetable or fish broth. Don't fry fish if you can help it—it's the least healthy method of cooking and adds unnecessary calories.

THINK FISH WHEN EATING OUT. Sushi is a great source of fish that is high in D. And many high-end restaurants serve oysters or shrimp as appetizers. Salmon is available on most menus, too. If you'd rather not cook fish yourself, ordering it when you dine out is a great way to enjoy this key D food and make it a regular part of your diet.

DAIRY

Most of the D experts I've interviewed over the years tell me that they prefer to get their D through milk. Most of them have a glass with every meal.

And they do this for good reason.

Dairy is one of many D-fortified foods, but it may very well rank as the most slimming of all your D-fortified options. Most types of dairy will net you about 100 IU of D per serving. In addition to being fortified with D, dairy is also rich in calcium, another important fat burner that I've already mentioned. Adequate levels of calcium help to reduce levels of fat storage hormones.

But the benefits don't stop there. Dairy is also rich in the amino acid leucine, which is important to stimulating muscle growth and fat burning. A review article published in the *Journal of the American College of Nutrition* found that leucine helps to protect lean muscle tissue and promote fat loss during dieting. It also helps to stabilize blood sugar levels.

Finally, the type of protein in dairy—whey protein—may help to reduce appetite above and beyond other types of protein. In one study by the US Department of Agriculture's Human Nutrition Research Center, women who consumed whey protein shakes along with their normal diets lost 2 pounds over 6 months and shrunk their waistlines—even though they were not dieting or trying to lose weight. Women who consumed carbohydrate shakes gained 2 pounds over the same time period, and women who consumed soy protein shakes maintained their weight.

This might be why dairy sources of calcium are twice as effective at promoting weight loss as calcium supplements, says Dr. Zemel, who has spent many years studying dairy, calcium, and weight loss at the University of Tennessee. The D, leucine, peptides, calcium, and other nutrients work together to boost weight loss and make milk and other fortified dairy products perfect weight-loss tools.

CONSUME THE DAIRY MINUS THE FAT. Because it's fortified, fat-free milk contains just as much D as its heavier cousins. It also provides plenty of protein and calcium, but with fewer calories.

OPT FOR A MILK ALTERNATIVE IF YOU CAN'T DO DAIRY. Although they lack some of the other weight-loss benefits of dairy (from the whey, peptides, and leucine), many varieties of soy milk, almond milk, and other milk substitutes are fortified with both D and calcium. Check the list of recommended brands in the Appendix for good options.

READ LABELS. All milk is fortified with 100 IU of D per serving, but yogurt and other dairy sources are hit-or-miss. Some brands of yogurt are fortified with as much as 30 percent of the DV per 6-ounce serving, whereas others contain none at all. This is also true of breakfast cereal, orange juice, and other fortified foods. Check labels to make the best choice. Use the label reading tips in the Appendix as well as the extensive list of recommended brands.

USE YOGURT AS A SAUCE, IN PLACE OF CREAM. A cup of D-fortified yogurt contains 80 IU of D. Mix 1 cup vitamin D–fortified plain yogurt with half a grated cucumber, 2 teaspoons of chopped fresh dill, 1 minced clove of garlic, 1 tablespoon of lemon juice, and salt and pepper to taste for a sauce that tastes great on top of fish.

USE DAIRY TO PUMP UP SMOOTHIES. The 7-Day Slim Down includes several delicious smoothie recipes for a reason. It's easy to pack multiple high-D foods into one smoothie. For instance, when you puree a handful of berries with 1 cup of D-fortified kefir or yogurt, you end up with 100 IU of D, plus several other slimmers. Top your smoothies with cinnamon, which will work along with D to help control blood sugar and insulin levels. The smoothie recipes are also loaded with fiber and protein to drive down appetite and keep you satisfied.

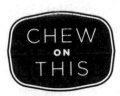

In the past, experts warned us against eating too many eggs, as the yolks are rich in both cholesterol and fat. That advice, however, is now outdated. Many studies show that egg yolks provide a wealth of good nutrition. Not only are they rich in D, they also house important antioxidants that improve your health— even your heart health.

EGGS

Studies suggest that eating protein in the morning will keep your hunger in check longer than eating a bagel or other high-carb foods, and eggs are a great way to get that protein. One egg has only 75 calories but packs 7 grams of high-quality protein, along with other vital nutrients.

In addition to providing appetite-suppressing protein, eggs are also one of nature's few natural sources of D. They contain other important slim-mers as well, including omega-3s (found in the yolk) and leucine, the same amino acid that I mentioned earlier and is also found in dairy.

PICK FREE-RANGE OR OMEGA EGGS, NOT CONVENTIONAL EGGS: Eggland's Best and other "omega" eggs come from hens who consume a special diet that yields eggs that are higher in D. The eggs contain 80 IU of D per egg, compared to just 40 IU for a conventional egg. And although researchers have not compared free-range eggs with those from conventionally raised chickens, it makes sense that hens exposed to sunlight would have more naturally circulating D that would eventually make its way into their eggs. A com-parison by *Mother Earth News* found that eggs from free-range hens had six times more D than eggs from conventional hens.

MAKE THE MOST OF HARD-COOKED EGGS. I like to make a batch or two at the beginning of each week. If you are anything like me, you probably don't particularly like the yolk, which can become quite dry if you hard-cook the egg according to most standard instructions. That's why I slightly underboil my eggs. This allows me to create an egg that has a cooked-through center that is moist and soft—not hard and flaky. To make eggs like mine, add the eggs to boiling water. Remove them after 9½ to 10 minutes. Place them immediately in a bath of ice water until they are completely cool.

MUSHROOMS

Mushrooms naturally contain only small amounts of D, but that's mostly because, until recently, all of them were grown and harvested in darkness. Not long ago, however, scientists realized that mushrooms can use sunlight to make D in much the same way humans do in their skin. When mushrooms are exposed to UVB light from fluo-rescent bulbs just before packaging, their D levels jump dramatically.

Regular mushrooms harvested in darkness have 6 to 10 IU of D per 3 ounces. One harvested in UVB light has close to 600 IU. The mushrooms lose some of that D during the first 3 days after expo-sure, so food manufacturers estimate that 3 ounces of most high-D mushrooms contain about 400 IU by the time they make their way to your kitchen.

In addition to D, mushrooms can help you lose weight for several additional reasons, starting with the fact that they are super low in calories. This allows you to consume a large volume—and thus fill up your stomach—without gaining weight. This makes mushrooms a great way to extend other foods, such as ground beef. Study participants who consumed mushrooms rather than meat, for

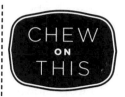

For easier-to-peel eggs, hard-cook eggs that are a few days old—not fresh. Eggs lose carbon dioxide through their shells as they age, which shrinks the egg inside the shell, creating a convenient little air pocket between the egg and the shell. When you hard-cook an older egg, this air pocket makes it easier to remove the shell without destroying the egg.

instance, shed nearly 13 pounds over 5 weeks. In a separate study done at Johns Hopkins University, researchers asked more than 50 participants to eat either mushroom- or meat-based lunches for 4 days. The mushroom-based lunches were of similar portion size but contained a lot fewer calories. People who consumed the mushroom lunches did not report increased hunger even though they consumed 444 fewer calories during their mushroom meals.

CHECK THE LABEL. Not all mushrooms are high in D, but most that are have a sticker with a high-D claim. On the nutrition facts label on the package, high-D mushrooms are listed as containing 100 percent of the DV for D, which translates to 400 IU.

DO SOME SLEUTHING. At the time this book was written, only two companies were making and marketing high-D mushrooms. You'll find more information about these companies in the Appendix. It's my hope that high-D mushrooms become more widely available around the country. At the moment, one of these companies, Monterey Mushrooms, sells these high-D mushrooms in most parts of the country at Kroger, Walmart, Whole Foods Market, and several other chains. Their button, crimini, and portobello mushrooms contain at least 400 IU per 3-ounce serving. If D-rich mushrooms are not available in your grocery store, you can find them online.

Mushrooms are higher in protein than most people think, making them a great food choice for vegetarians. They are also rich in fiber, which suppresses appetite and helps you fill up on fewer calories. And certain types of mushrooms are packed with antioxidants, which are good for your overall health.

STORE THEM CORRECTLY. You want to keep mushrooms dry, so don't wash them until just before using them. Either keep them in a paper bag in the fridge or in their original packaging.

COOK THEM. Cooking does not destroy or remove any of the D, but it does remove the water, concentrating the nutrients per serving.

Usually you don't want to make a food more dense, but mushrooms are so low in calories that this isn't an issue. Cooking them can allow you to quadruple the D in each serving. Here's an easy way to make them and use them as a topping for other foods: Spread sliced mushrooms and onions on a baking sheet. Drizzle with good quality balsamic vinegar. Roast at 350°F until the mushrooms are lightly browned and glazed. Toss with chopped parsley or sprinkle with a little sea salt.

CHOOSE DRIED MUSHROOMS, TOO. A serving of sun-dried shiitake mushrooms contains a whopping 1,600 IU of vitamin D! Just follow package directions to soak them. They will absorb the water, soften, and return to the texture of a fresh mushroom.

WHOLE GRAIN BREAD

More and more brands of bread are now fortified with D and sometimes even with calcium, too.

This is great because bread, especially whole grain bread, offers many weight-loss benefits. Penn State researchers have found that the consumption of whole grains is associated with lower body weight. In a Penn State study, 50 people who chose products with a whole grain listed as the first ingredient lost more weight in the tummy region than participants who consumed refined grains.

Dieters who consume whole grains also better maintain their weight loss. Bran is a particularly powerful whole grain option, seeming to prevent regain more than other types of grains do.

Whole grain bread is also a rich source of fiber, and fiber helps to reduce appetite. A Brigham Young University study of 252 women determined that for every 1-gram increase in fiber consumption, body weight decreased by half a pound. (The study spanned 20 months.) Depending on the type of bread you purchase, you can benefit from two types of fiber.

INSOLUBLE FIBER: This is the type of fiber that stays intact and bulks up the contents in your intestines so your stool gets heavy, slippery, and easy to pass. In other words, it keeps you regular and in and out of the bathroom quickly—no reading material required. It's found in whole grains, fruits, vegetables, and bran.

SOLUBLE FIBER: This type of fiber tends to grab onto the starch, fat, and cholesterol in your food, mixing with these food components to form a viscous, slow-moving gel. As fiber mixes with food, it may thwart some of the food calories from ever getting absorbed into your bloodstream and slow the absorption of others. This type of fiber also ferments in the colon, which provides some health benefits. It's found in fruits, vegetables, oats, legumes, and seeds.

READ LABELS. Just because bread is brown in color doesn't mean it contains whole grains. Purchase bread that lists a whole grain flour first on the list of ingredients, such as "whole wheat flour" or "100% whole wheat flour." Food manufacturers are required by law to list ingredients in descending order of how much they weigh. So the most prevalent and heaviest ingredients are listed first. Ideally, choose bread that has 2 grams or more of fiber per slice. You'll find recommended bread brands that are both whole grain and high in D in the Appendix.

LOOK FOR A WHOLE GRAIN SEAL. If it has a seal on the front of the package that says "whole grain," that means at least 51 percent of the ingredients are whole grains by weight.

TOFU

Tofu is one of the star D foods because not only is it fortified, it's what makes high-D eating truly possible for vegetarians. Although other key D foods can be incorporated into a vegetarian diet, tofu offers a strong source of D, calcium, and protein.

Even without the fortification, tofu is a great weight-loss food because it's high in protein and low in calories. A ½ cup adds up to only 88 calories but provides 1 gram of fiber and 10 grams of protein. That's a huge fiber and protein punch for so few calories—making tofu an incredibly filling food.

It's also a versatile food that can be a great substitute for calorie-laden fatty spreads like mayo. And you can use it to extend high-calorie foods. For instance, combine ground beef with tofu and mushrooms when making burgers to cut down on some of the beef and fill up on fewer calories. And you can even add it to smoothies to help fill up on fewer calories.

READ LABELS. Not all tofu is high in D. Consult the list of recommended foods in the Appendix to find brands that are.

USE TOFU AS A SUBSTITUTE FOR MAYO. Combine 16 ounces of silken tofu with ½ ounce of sugar, ½ ounce of cornstarch, and lemon juice, vinegar, dry mustard, salt, and cayenne to taste. Or you can puree it in a blender with lemon juice, salt, pepper, and a little cheese and use it as a substitute for sour cream.

USE TOFU AS A LOW-CALORIE FOOD EXTENDER. Mix it into ground beef. Add silken tofu to creamy spreads and dips.

MASTER SIMPLE COOKING TECHNIQUES. If you aren't a fan of tofu's consistency, there are easy ways to make it more of a "burger" patty or a faux meat. Drain tofu of excess water by placing a plate or something heavy on top of it until you've squeezed most of the water out of it. Then marinate it, slice it into ½-inch slices, and bake for 30 minutes at 375°F. Broil for a few minutes on each side before serving.

ORANGE JUICE

Orange juice is sometimes fortified with both D and calcium, making it a great way to boost the D content of your morning meal. It's also rich in vitamin C, which may also aid weight loss. A study done at Arizona State University found that people with higher blood levels of C had smaller waistlines than people with lower blood levels.

There are no do's and don'ts to suggest here because OJ is so simple. Enjoy a glass a day for a 100-IU boost in D. You can drink it alone or add it to smoothies. Check the list of recommended brands in the Appendix to find D-fortified OJ. Use the menus and recipes for serving suggestions.

WHOLE GRAIN BREAKFAST CEREAL

Breakfast cereal—both hot and cold—rounds out the list of star foods. Like bread, breakfast cereals can be rich sources of whole grains and fiber, making them great appetite suppressors.

Studies find that people who eat cereal for breakfast every day are significantly less likely to be obese than those who don't. They also consume more fiber and calcium—and less fat—than those who eat other breakfast foods.

My best tip for cereal is this: Consider eating it for lunch and dinner, too, or after a workout. A bowl of cereal is an easy meal to eat when you are on the run or just too tired to cook. Once you add milk, you are pumping up the D even more. And if you add a glass of OJ to the mix, your total D content for that meal can top 300 IU. For variety, consider mixing cereal in with D-fortified yogurt, rather than milk.

Make sure you pick a brand that is high in fiber, fortified with D, and low in sugar. You'll find several recommended brands in the Appendix.

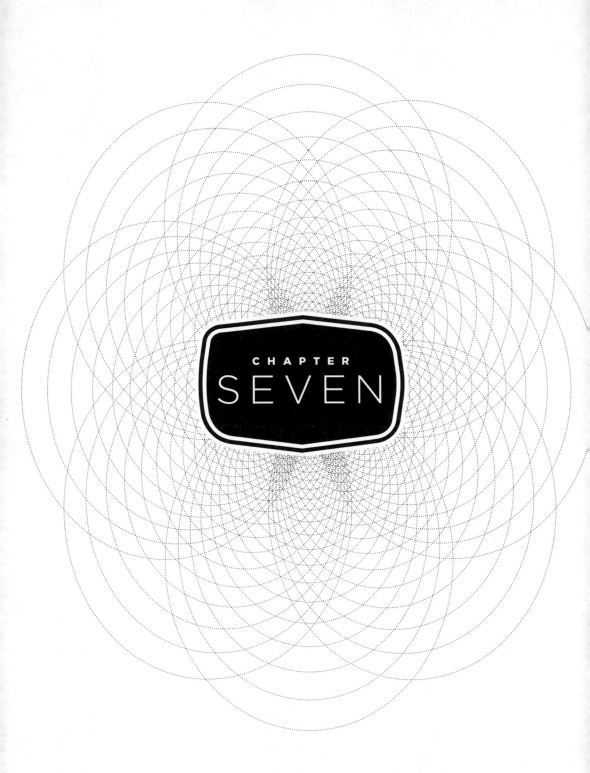

CHAPTER
SEVEN

How You'll Achieve Success

Y ou've read the scientific support for the 7-Day Slim Down. You've seen the studies, you've heard from the experts, and you've read about the historical evidence. You know why it works, and you know how soon it will work. Now it's time for you to get results. It's time to slim down!

The rules in the following pages will teach you how to follow the 7-Day Slim Down for immediate and lasting weight loss—for the rest of your life. The tips and advice are memorable, easy to follow, and customizable to fit your lifestyle. Can you make substitutions? Absolutely. Can you drink alcohol or eat out? Yes, and yes, and the advice for doing both is realistic and sensible.

Five Steps to a Slimmer, Healthier You

YOU'LL LOSE WEIGHT on this plan by following five easy steps.

1 DETERMINE YOUR D PROFILE. Before you embark on the actual diet, you need to get a sense of your D status. I'm going to wager that you are either sub-optimal or deficient. Chapter 8 will help you make this assessment. Based on your results, you'll find out whether you need to take a D supplement only in the winter, whether you should stay on your supplement year-round, or whether you really ought to work with a physician to determine the best D dose for you.

2 START THE 7-DAY SLIM DOWN. Once you have determined your profile, you are ready to drop pounds in record time.

In Chapter 9, you will find a week's worth of detailed and specific menus. These menus will help you to optimize your D, superdosing your body with roughly 1,000 IU of D a day. This, plus your supplement and any sunlight you might be getting, will give you a jump start on replenishing those D stores so you can speed weight loss along—losing up to 7 pounds in the first week.

3 **PROGRESS TO THE 4-WEEK SLIM DOWN.** Once the 7-Day Slim Down has primed you with D and jump-started your weight loss, you're ready for the main eating plan. This is where you gain flexibility and can create your own supercharged meals and menus. You'll find 4 weeks' worth of mix-and-match options for breakfast, lunch, and dinner—all of which make it easy for you to consume 600 IU of D or more a day, along with the right amount of calcium, too. Even though this plan is called The 4-Week Slim Down, it's designed so that you'll have plenty of options so you can stay on the plan until you've reached your weight-loss goals. Then, you'll adapt the maintenance plan to fit your needs so that you can stick to it for life.

4 **USE THE SEASONAL PLANS, DEPENDING ON THE TIME OF YEAR.** It doesn't make sense to eat the same way in the winter as you do in the summer. In the winter, your body craves hot, stick-to-your-ribs meals. In the summer, it's the opposite. You also need more D in the winter than you do in the summer. That's why I created a summer and a winter plan that you can incorporate into the main eating plan as needed.

5 **EMBARK ON THE MAINTENANCE SLIM DOWN.** Once you reach your weight-loss goal, it's time to shift into maintenance mode. You'll find everything you need to know about keeping the pounds off and staying slim for good in Chapter 15.

Seven Rules for Lasting Success

NO MATTER WHICH part of the plan you are on at any given time, make sure you abide by the following rules—they're the keys to lasting weight loss and the slimmer, sexier body you desire. These rules are meant to fit into even the busiest, most challenging schedules and lifestyles. They've worked for real women—and they'll work for you too.

RULE #1

WATCH YOUR PORTIONS

As I've mentioned, this plan optimizes D, calcium, and other nutrients to help you melt fat fast. That said, if you eat more calories than your body burns, you won't be able to lose much weight. It's just as important to consume the correct portions as it is to get enough D and other slimmers.

The menus in *The 7-Day Slim Down* are all specifically calculated to fuel your body with roughly 1,400 to 1,500 daily calories. This number of calories will shift your body into weight-loss mode without triggering age-old starvation mechanisms that turn up hunger and slow metabolism. If you consume the right portions suggested by the plan, you will experience steady weight loss until you reach your goal.

Measure your portions, especially in the beginning. Research shows that most people underestimate what they eat by anywhere from 20 to 200 percent. That's a lot, and this portion distortion can easily slow, stop, or even reverse your weight loss. To avoid it, measuring devices are in order. Get out the measuring cups and spoons. Over time, you'll be able to eyeball portions. In the beginning, however, don't trust your eyes. Trust your tools instead. Once you plate your food, take a look at it and memorize what the correct portion looks like. Eventually, test yourself. Plate your food and then quickly measure it to see how close you were to correctly eyeballing the portion. Once you can eyeball the portion accurately, you can move away from the measuring devices.

Learn a few tricks of the portion control trade. If you compare portions to objects from real life, you'll gain a better sense of the correct size and shape of the portion you are attempting to plate. A $1/2$ cup of cooked grains, for instance, is roughly the size of a tennis ball. One cup of pasta (2 ounces) or cereal (1 ounce) is the size of your fist. A cup of veggies is the size of a baseball. A $1/2$ cup of fruit or veggies is the size of a lightbulb. A quarter cup is the size of an egg. One and a half ounces of cheese is roughly the size of a 9-volt battery. Three ounces of meat is the size of a checkbook or a deck of cards.

When in doubt, plate more vegetables and dairy. Most people eat fewer veggies and less dairy than they think, so be sure to load up your plate with greens and healthy milk and cheese options. They'll fill you up so you feel satisfied and don't overdo it on the fats and sweets.

Only serve what you are planning to eat. Your eyes are a window to your stomach. The more food you see, the hungrier you feel. The less food you see, the less hungry you feel. It may sound obvious, but studies show that if you serve people more food, they'll eat more food. The converse is also true: Serve yourself less and you'll automatically want to eat less. This is especially important in restaurants. Ask the waitstaff to bring you a half portion, rather than attempting to halve it for yourself at the table.

RULE #2

USE THE 90/10 PRINCIPLE

It's my philosophy that a diet that conflicts with having a life isn't a diet that is worth following. And, unfortunately, that's exactly what many diets do. Who wants to be sitting there with a protein drink when everyone else is enjoying a buffet of hot food? It's also quite difficult to have a life if you can't occasionally eat birthday cake or a big pasta dinner, or whatever your favorite indulgent meal might be.

A diet only works if you can follow it long-term. And you can only follow a diet long-term if you are able to make little tweaks, nips, and tucks that seamlessly fit that plan into your life. That's where the 90/10 principle comes in. According to this principle, you will follow the 7-Day Slim Down 90 percent of the time. The other 10 percent of the time, you eat what you want—within reason.

I say within reason because many people have misinterpreted the 90/10 rule over the years. I have a friend who thought it meant that she should follow a diet to a T during the week and then eat what-ever she wanted on weekends. Well, let me tell you, her weekends were huge gorge fests, and they completely undid all of the hard work she'd put in during the week. Worse, they worked to unravel her resolve. Her weekend gorge kept starting a little earlier and lasting a little longer. Before she knew it, she was gorging 90 per-cent of the time and dieting 10 percent of the time. Eventually, she wasn't dieting at all!

So that's what the 90/10 principle *isn't*. Let's take a closer look at what the 90/10 principle is.

Never forget Rule #1. To successfully put the 90/10 principle to work for you, you must do one thing as consistently as you can. Always practice Rule #1: portion control. As long as you do that, you can stay on this plan no matter what the situation. For instance, let's say you want your aunt's mouthwatering stuffing

on Thanksgiving. No problem. Just calculate a 400-calorie portion for yourself, and enjoy every bite. Or let's say you have had one of those days and all you want to do is rent a movie and eat popcorn laced with M&M's all night long. Feel free to indulge! Again, just do so consciously—portion out 400 calories' worth of popcorn and M&Ms and put the rest away. The principle works the same for your vitamin D consumption, as well. If 90 percent of your meals are high in D and 10 percent of them are not, you'll still come out ahead.

Don't stray too far or for too long. Remember the story about my friend? Her weekend gorges were problematic because they gradually worked to derail her weight-loss efforts completely. Remember this rule of physics: An object in motion tends to stay in motion. You overcame a lot of inertia in order to start this plan. Don't lose your momentum! Be wary of taking a 2-week break or even a weekend-long break from the plan. Usually, extended breaks are when the weight starts creeping back. Once you've adjusted to the meal plan, an occasional indulgence should be enough to make you feel as though you've had a special treat.

Pop a supplement. Use it as insurance on your low-D days. If you normally take 1,000 IU, boost it up to 2,000 IU.

Use 90/10 when eating out, too. This plan encourages you to enjoy your favorite restaurants. That said, restaurant food generally contains an addictive combination of flavors (usually sweet plus salty) and ingredients (usually butter, salt, and sugar) that makes it hard to stay in control. It's also hard to ensure you are getting the right foods when you order. Most restaurants, for instance, still use refined grain products that are low in fiber or mushrooms that are not high in D. You can still lose weight while eating out, but you'll lose it faster and keep it off more easily if you prepare 90 percent of your meals at home.

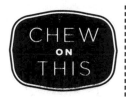

CHEW ON THIS

When your body lacks calcium, it can experience up to a fivefold increase in the fatty acid synthase, an enzyme that converts calories into fat. In a 2009 study published in the British Journal of Nutrition, obese women who were put on a 15-week diet and took 1,200 milligrams of calcium lost six times more weight than women who followed the diet alone.

RULE #3

COUNT YOUR IU OF D

On some plans you count carbs. On others, you count fat grams.

On this plan, I'd like you to count IUs, especially in the beginning. Short for International Unit, an IU is simply a unit of measurement. In this case, it's measuring vitamin D.

In addition to your IUs of D, I'd also like you to keep track of your milligrams of calcium. That's because D and calcium are the two power nutrients on this plan, and they work synergistically to help you melt fat. Both nutrients work to speed fat burning, but you really can't benefit from one without having optimal amounts of the other. Vitamin D is critical to enabling the body to absorb calcium. A person who is vitamin D deficient will absorb only one-third as much calcium as he or she would with healthy vitamin D levels. And I've mentioned, studies at the University of Tennessee and Purdue University show that diets high in calcium lead to the release of a hormone that turns up fat burning. Upping calcium and vitamin D intake while reducing calories forces your body to convert fat into fuel—and shed pounds.

Change your goal depending on the time of year. You need more D in the winter than you do in the summer. During the summer months, you're probably getting some D from sunlight, so you can drop the amount you get from food to about 600 IU a day. During the winter, however,

it's best to bump that goal up to 1,000 IU. Your calcium requirement is always the same: 1,000 milligrams a day.

	WINTER	SUMMER
VITAMIN D GOAL	1,000 IU	600 IU
CALCIUM GOAL	1,000 mg	1,000 mg

Use the menus as a guide. I've included the D and calcium amounts on every single menu option. Most are high enough in both nutrients that you will be hard-pressed to create menus for yourself that dip below 600 IU for D and 1,000 milligrams for calcium. Still, it's a good idea to jot down total D and calcium levels as you go so you can see how you are doing.

Pick the right foods. As you progress on the plan, you will eventually create your own D- and calcium-rich meals. If you eat three D-rich foods and three calcium-rich foods a day, you will automatically come close to meeting your requirements.

RULE #4
TAKE A SUPPLEMENT
I'd love to tell you that you can get all the D you need from natural food sources and from the sun. But the truth is, you may need some assistance from another source. Spending too much time in the sun without adequate skin protection causes everything from early wrinkles to melanoma. And there aren't enough D-rich foods for you to easily consume adequate levels of D. I say easily because sure, you could eat wild salmon topped with mushrooms every single day. But I'm certainly not willing to do that, and I doubt you are, either.

That's why a supplement is in order. The good news is that D supplements are cheap, easy to find, and easy to swallow. (I've never been able to choke down the average multivitamin. They are just too large and tend to tickle my gag reflex!)

D supplements are usually small, smooth capsules that are pain-less to swallow. Follow these guidelines when you go shopping.

Base your dosage on your D Profile. You will calculate your D profile in the next chapter, but here's a general suggestion. If you are obese or have more than 20 pounds to lose, take a supple-ment year-round and aim for 2,000 IU daily. If you have fewer than 10 to 20 pounds to lose, take a supplement at least during the winter months—November through April—and opt for a lower dosage of 1,000 IU. I recommend that you get your D levels tested once a year—preferably during the winter. You can do this as part of your annual cholesterol screening, and it's often covered by insurance.

Take a supplement even if you are already taking a multivitamin. Most multivitamins only contain 400 IU of D or less. That's just not enough.

Don't worry about toxicity. As I've mentioned, the risk of toxicity doesn't kick in until you've gone way over the amounts I'm sug-gesting in this book. All of the vitamin D experts I interviewed take a D supplement (usually 2,000 IU) with a multivitamin, and many also drink three glasses of milk a day. They average 2,700 IU of D a day, and that doesn't include sun exposure. They all recom-mended this strategy to others regardless of their geographic location, weight, or race.

Don't lean on the supplement too much. It's still important to follow a D-rich diet. You'll never lose weight by taking a pill and not changing anything else about your diet. And remember: Food contains many nutrients that just can't be easily extracted and packaged into pills. The 4-Week Slim Down menus will do more than merely fuel your body with an optimal daily dose of D. They will also prime you with all of the nutrients you need to switch into fat-melting mode and stay there.

RULE #5

DIET FIRST, EXERCISE WHEN YOU ARE READY

Exercise is an important ingredient to weight-loss success. It's certainly a component of this plan, as I outline in Chapter 14. But it's important to understand that while exercise is very important for weight loss and your overall health, you don't necessarily need to incorporate it into your diet plan from the very beginning. In fact, people often find it easier and more enjoyable to exercise after they've already lost some weight, as opposed to starting an exercise program before they've shed some pounds.

Be true to yourself. If you are the kind of person who is super motivated and quite capable of accomplishing a lot of change at once, then it might be best to start your fitness program now, when you are most motivated to tackle change. On the other hand, if you are the type of person who prefers to ease into change slowly, then work on learning the diet first. Get used to the recipes and get the meal plan down. Then, once everything feels familiar to you, tackle the exercise plan. Choose what you know you will be able to accomplish so you don't get frustrated and set yourself up for failure.

Consider your body size. If you are very overweight, you'll find an exercise plan a lot easier to tackle once you've lost a few pounds. It's a lot more comfortable to move a smaller body than it is to move a larger one. Perhaps even more important, once you bring D levels back up to optimal, you'll be more likely to feel like moving, too. When D levels are below normal, you feel it in your bones and in your muscles. Everything aches. By dieting first and exercising second, you can bring D levels up, reduce that achiness, and start off your exercise program on the right foot.

Do what you love. You'll hear this advice from me over and over again. If you force yourself to do a fitness routine that you hate just because you know it will burn a lot of calories, you won't be doing that fitness routine for long. The most important benefit you can get from exercise is increased muscle mass. It doesn't take a high degree of intensity to reap that benefit. Do just enough, but don't overdo it and burn yourself out. Find the sweet spot.

Bring some light into your fitness routine. The best exercise you can do, both for your fat cells and your mood, is an exercise you can do outdoors. Even in the winter, when the sun's angle is too low to help you replenish your D stores, outdoor exercise will still boost mood and energy and help to reduce cravings, too.

RULE #6

EAT BY THE SEASONS

Your body needs different nutrients, flavors, and textures in the winter than it does in the summer. Most notably, it needs more D. But, if your body is like mine, it also craves heavier, heartier foods in the winter. The last thing I want is a salad or smoothie. No, I want something with heft and warmth—like stew or chili or soup.

And in the summer, it's the opposite. Lighter fare is in order. During the summer you also need less D from food because you'll be getting at least some of your D from sunlight. So you can ease up on salmon and other foods that are super high in D and gravitate toward more salads and smoothies and other light fare.

Use the 4-Week Slim Down as your base. Then mix and match the Winter Warming Menus and the Summer Light Menus based on the time of year.

Create your own seasonal favorites. *The 7-Day Slim Down* menus provide you with formulas for making your own signature soups, stews, salads, and smoothies.

Switch from one plan to another based on where you live. In some parts of the world, winter starts earlier and lasts longer. If you live in the southern United States, you might want to stay on the summer plan until late November, or perhaps even into December. If you live in Alaska, you'll probably want to switch to the winter plan much earlier. Let your body be your guide. It will tell you when it wants to switch. Trust me. Suddenly you'll get a hankering for beef stew, and you'll think, "Must be time for the winter warming menus."

RULE #7

BE SUN SMART

When I first began pulling together research and interviews for this book, I was a devoted believer in the American Academy of Dermatology's recommendation on sun exposure, which is this: No amount of unprotected sun exposure is safe. The Academy recommends you wear a broad-spectrum sunscreen of SPF 30 or higher whenever you are outdoors, no matter the season or time of day. In addition, the Academy recommends you take steps to stay out of the sun whenever possible by wearing a broad-brimmed hat or standing in the shade.

After all, no one wants to get skin cancer—a problem that affects one in five people. No woman wants to get wrinkles, age spots, or skin discoloration, either.

But some of my research was confusing. When I interviewed Dr. Holick of Boston University, he told me that the sun is our best source of vitamin D. Our skin makes D faster and in higher amounts than anything we could consume from food alone or even from high-dose supplements. Just 30 to 60 minutes on a beach in a swimsuit during the height of summer will net you close to 20,000 IU of D. And that D will stay active in your body longer than D from food or supplements will.

For a short while after learning this, I was quite lax at protecting myself from the sun. I wore sunscreen when I knew I would be outdoors for a long period of time. But if I was just going out for a 20-minute walk? I didn't bother.

Then my running partner was diagnosed with skin cancer. She underwent a procedure that involved extensive facial surgery and had to keep her face bandaged for weeks. (She's not a vain person at all, but the procedure made her extremely self-con- scious. I think anyone would feel the same.) While my running partner doesn't exactly sunbathe on a regular basis, she does run outdoors regularly. She's also had her D tested. It's in the normal range.

People who are deficient in D tend to have a higher risk for skin and other cancers. Getting your D into the optimal range might just be the best thing you can do to prevent cancer of any kind—even skin cancer. But even someone who has normal levels of D—much like my friend—can still be at risk for skin cancer and other sun- related problems. My friend's experience made me realize how important sun protection really is.

Always protect your face. This is the area of your body that is most exposed to the sun and most prone to premature aging and disfiguring cancers. Choose a daily moisturizer with a high SPF (ideally SPF 30) and reapply it throughout the day. For added benefit, you can also use mineral makeup, a special type of makeup made from minerals. Sold online and in spas, it naturally protects your skin from sunlight. If you will be outdoors for an extended period of time, apply stand-alone sunscreen of 30 SPF or higher. If you will be sweating or swimming, use a waterproof version, and always reapply after swimming no matter what type of sunscreen you are wearing.

Wear a hat. You can't protect your face enough. When you will be outdoors for an extended period of time, wear a wide-brimmed hat or a baseball cap to shade your face from the sun.

Consider safe exposure. The largest surface areas of your body that can soak up D from the sun (while you're still otherwise clothed) are your back, arms, and legs. But only do this for short periods of time—never more then 15 minutes a day. Keep your sunscreen-free time shorter if you are very light skinned and prone to burning.

Reapply often. Reapply sunscreen often, and especially after swimming, even if your sunscreen is waterproof.

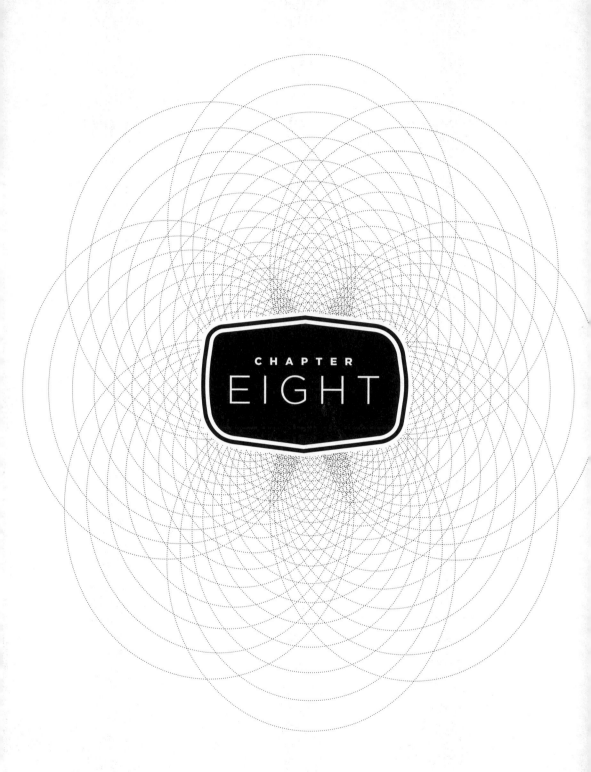

CHAPTER

EIGHT

Determine Your D Profile

My good friend Carole had been experiencing strange symptoms for months. She was unbelievably tired. Her muscles ached. And no matter what she did, she couldn't seem to lose weight.

Like many people, she'd initially suspected the worst: cancer. But that was quickly ruled out as well as other autoimmune diseases. She was tested for chronic pain conditions like fibromyalgia and chronic fatigue syndrome, too. She didn't have them. She didn't have a sleep disorder, either. Carole was starting to wonder if her physicians thought she was crazy and that her symptoms were all in her head.

"Would you believe they finally found out what's wrong with me?" Carole announced one day, with a great sense of triumph. "I have a vitamin D deficiency," she said.

At the time, I was already working on this book and doing a lot of writing on the topic. I'd seen the statistics about the high percentage of people with D deficiency. I'd already interviewed Dr. Holick, who had explained that more people were deficient than ever.

Still, I was shocked to hear Carole's news. For starters, she lived in Virginia and had a vacation home on the Chesapeake. She seemed to spend quite a bit of time in the sun. She is also of Irish descent and has pale skin; the kind that soaks up lots of sunlight in record time. Carole is the kind of person I would expect to tell me that she has skin cancer and needs to have half of her nose taken off. Frankly, she was the skin cancer type, not the vitamin D–deficiency type.

"Do you wear sunscreen religiously?" I asked.

"No, not really. Just when we're out on the boat," she replied.

As it turned out, Carole didn't have a single risk factor for D deficiency. Still, she was unbelievably deficient, and her doctor had her on high doses of D to correct that deficiency. "I'm feeling so much better!" she said. Indeed, as her D levels came up to normal, the mysterious aches and pains went away. So did the fatigue. And her weight began dropping, too.

A whopping 77 percent of all Americans are now vitamin D deficient, according to the National Health and Nutrition Examination Surveys (NHANES), published in the *Archives of Internal Medicine*. Are you one of them? Let's find out.

TEST YOUR
D STATUS

If you answer any of the following questions with a "yes,"
you might be D deficient and should ask your doctor for a
25 (OH) D test (25-hydroxyvitamin D test).
With every "yes" answer, your risk of deficiency goes up.

○ DO YOU WORK INDOORS?

○ DO YOU WEAR SUNSCREEN RELIGIOUSLY?

○ DO YOU LIVE IN AN AIR-POLLUTED LOCATION?

○ ARE YOU A PERSON OF COLOR?

○ ARE YOU OVERWEIGHT OR OBESE?

○ DO YOU LIVE NORTH OF ATLANTA?

RISK FACTOR #1:
YOU WORK INDOORS

As I mentioned earlier, our hunter-gatherer ancestors evolved in sunlight. And even as little as 100 years ago, our ancestors spent most of the day outdoors in the sun as they worked on farms and performed other outdoor activities. Spending all day sitting inside at your desk is a fairly recent phenomenon. And now, with the world economy in such bad shape, people are working longer and longer hours inside.

To manufacture enough D from sunlight, you need to be in the sun at a time of day that many of us just aren't. Our skin makes little D before 9 a.m. and after 4 p.m., says Dr. Holick.

"Most of us are working longer and longer hours to make ends meet. This means that you step through the office door before sunrise and leave after sunset, especially during the winter months, when days are shorter," says Roberta Anding, MS, RD, sports dietitian for the Houston Texans and Astros.

If you rarely see the sun, chances are, you're deficient.

YOU WEAR SUNSCREEN RELIGIOUSLY

Ideally, you would get your D from the sun. After all, that's what our ancestors did, and it's what our bodies are genetically designed to do. When your skin makes its own vitamin D, the vitamin lasts twice as long in your blood as when you eat the vitamin or get it through a supplement. Even if you manage to get outdoors during peak hours (10 a.m. to 3 p.m.), you need to expose more than just your face to the sun in order to make enough D. Your face just doesn't have enough surface area to soak up enough rays and make enough D to supply your body with all the D it needs.

Yet, with the exception of the summer months, most of us wear clothes—long sleeve shirts and long skirts or pants—that make it difficult for our skin to make any D, even when we are outdoors in the sunlight. Makeup—especially mineral makeup—also blocks D. And so does sunscreen, which reduces your skin's ability to make D by 90 to 99 percent, depending on the SPF. So even during the summer months when you are wearing a tank and shorts, you are probably not getting enough D if you are sun-smart and doing what dermatologists have been telling us to do ever since the hole in the ozone layer was discovered.

Dr. Holick has generated controversy by recommending what he calls "sensible sun exposure," which means exposing large areas of your body (especially your arms and legs) to the sun during peak hours (10 a.m. to 3 p.m.). Dr. Holick says you should do this without sunscreen for one quarter to half the time it would take for you to get a little pink. If you are very fair skinned, that's probably about 15 minutes. If you are darker skinned, it's closer to 2 hours. Other experts, like Dr. Norman, aren't as quick to recommend sun exposure as a way to get D. "There's no question that generous sun exposure over a lifetime does lead to skin cancer. We can't undo that," says Dr. Norman. "At the same time, Mother Nature did not intend for vitamin D to be a vitamin that we consume as a supplement. She intended for us to make it in our skin."

The American Academy of Dermatology says that there's no safe level of sunlight exposure. Their advice: Use sunscreen or other sun protection daily, skip the tanning booths, and get your vitamin D from diet or supplements.

Personally, I don't go into the sun without sunscreen. Two of my friends have already been diagnosed with skin cancer and had the tips of their noses removed as a result (seriously—scary!) Yes, plastic surgeons can work miracles. Still, having facial reconstructive surgery is a miracle I would rather not experience firsthand. My take: Keep up your sunscreen use, especially on your face. We should all be able to check off this risk factor, even if it means we're more D-ficient.

RISK FACTOR #3:

YOU LIVE IN AN AIR-POLLUTED CITY

Air pollution filters out some of the UVB rays, so fewer of them are able to reach your skin. This is one reason why folks who live in Los Angeles and Atlanta tend to be deficient despite their sunny, warm locations. Another possible reason might be that, in hotter climates, people are more likely to stay indoors with the AC on and to routinely use sunscreen.

If you are not sure if you live in an air-polluted location, you can check with the American Lung Association. It publishes a report each year that lists the most air-polluted cities. Ask for the "State of the Air" report, or search for it online.

YOU ARE A PERSON OF COLOR

Darker skin pigmentation makes it more difficult to generate vitamin D. The melanin in skin acts as a natural sunscreen that blocks rays from getting to your skin. The darker your skin, the higher your natural SPF and the more sunlight your skin needs to make D.

Eighty-four percent of African-Americans tested at Boston University were deficient in D, compared to 40 percent of Hispanics and 34 percent of Caucasians.

YOU ARE OVERWEIGHT OR OBESE

For many years, researchers have known that supplementing overweight and obese people with D doesn't produce the same results as supplementing the lean. A doctor can get a lean person's D levels up to normal fairly quickly with a low-dose supplement. But the heavier someone is, the more D it takes to get her blood levels up to normal. It takes roughly 50 percent more D to bring blood levels up to normal in the obese than it does in the lean.

Body fat hoards D, preventing it from getting into the bloodstream and to the tissues and cells that need it. D is a fat-soluble vitamin, which means that it prefers to hang out and be stored in your body fat. It doesn't like to hang out in watery substances like blood and most body tissues. So the more fat you have, the more places D has to hide and the less D is available for the tissues that desperately need it.

How do you figure out if you are actually obese? You'll want to calculate your Body Mass Index (BMI). This is simply a calculation of your weight and height. The actual formula looks a tad scary ([weight in pounds/height inches]^2 x 703)—but any number of online calculators can figure out your BMI for you as well as show you what range you fall into (underweight, normal, or overweight).

You can also download the BMI iPhone app from the National Heart, Lung, and Blood Institute.

A less scientific, but very simple test: Strip down to your underwear and jump up and down in front of a mirror. Nutrition expert Roberta Anding taught me this test, and I think it's genius (if a little cringe-worthy). "If it jiggles, it's from excess fat," she says. This excess fat means you might be D deficient.

RISK FACTOR #6:

YOU LIVE NORTH OF ATLANTA

If you sat out in a bathing suit on a sunny afternoon for long enough to turn your skin slightly pink, you could make plenty of vitamin D, but only during the summer months. During late autumn and winter at higher latitudes, the angle of the sun is too low for enough rays to get to your skin to create enough D. In fact, people who live at higher latitudes can't make any D during much of the year.

By higher latitudes you might think I'm talking about places like the Arctic Circle around Lapland, where the sun never shines during the winter months. I'm not. I'm talking about most places north of Atlanta.

Imagine a line cutting across the United States, starting at Atlanta and crossing through northern Alabama and Mississippi and continuing across the country until it reaches Los Angeles. If you live north of that line, your skin probably doesn't get enough sunlight to make D between November and March.

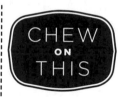

You must lose roughly 15 percent of your body weight before the D that is stored in your fat can be released and used. That's 30 pounds for a 200-pound woman. Women who lost more than 15 percent of their body weight saw a boost double that amount, according to research done at the Fred Hutchinson Cancer Research Center. Women who lost only 5 to 15 percent of their body weight saw a corresponding increase of only 2 to 3 ng/ml in D levels.

Get Your D Tested

IT'S QUITE POSSIBLE that you took the test above and didn't have a single risk factor mentioned in this chapter—but like my friend Carole, you could still be D deficient anyway. A blood test administered by a doctor is the most reliable way to tell not only whether you are deficient, but also how severe your deficiency is.

Make sure you get the correct test for D, as some doctors prescribe the wrong test, which can give you a false negative. The body goes to great lengths to maintain a steady level of active D in the blood, just as it does with calcium and other nutrients. In order to keep blood levels of active D steady, it will pull D from elsewhere in the body. It does the same with calcium. So the tissues that need D the most can be terribly low in it, even if your blood levels of active D are normal or even higher than normal.

The correct test is called a 25-hydroxyvitamin D test. It's also called a 25 (OH) D test. This is a test of your circulating, nonactive levels of D, and it will give you and your doctor an accurate sense of whether the various tissues in your body are lacking in D. Many internists now perform the D test routinely, as part of an annual cholesterol screening. If yours does, consider yourself ahead of the game. If yours doesn't, ask for the test. And you can strengthen your case if you have any of the risk factors described in this chapter.

In addition to getting the right test, it's also important to interpret the results correctly. There's a lot of controversy over what constitutes vitamin D deficiency. While the Institute of Medicine says that blood levels of D must be below 20 ng/ml for you to be considered deficient, other experts believe the target number should be higher. The Endocrine Society, for instance, recommends that you shoot for at least 30 ng/ml and ideally your level should fall between 40 and 60 ng/ml.

Why such a discrepancy?

"The Institute of Medicine is extremely cautious," says Dr. Norman who first discovered the D receptor on the intestines. "Their guidelines are based on what they think is good for bone health, but that doesn't solve the problem of what is good for your immune system, pancreas, muscles, heart muscle, and brain."

Or your fat cells.

So You're High Risk. Now What?

HERE'S THE THING with all of the questions I posed in this chapter. It's nearly impossible to not answer yes to at least one of them. I'm guessing most of you probably wear sunscreen, work indoors, or live north of Atlanta—or all three.

You almost can't take the test without having at least one risk factor, and most people have more than one. That's why so many people are deficient in D.

So get tested. Based on your results, your doctor will help you get your D levels up to normal. If you are severely deficient, your doctor will likely prescribe high-dose vitamin D supplements— somewhere between 5,000 and 10,000 IU. While it's not prudent to self-medicate with dosages that high without the supervision of a doctor, these high dosages can bring D levels up to normal quickly.

Now let's say you have one or more risk factors but you don't want to get your D tested by your doctor. I understand that blood tests are expensive and not everyone has health insurance. And not everyone has free time for

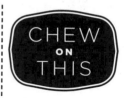

CHEW ON THIS

Vitamin D testing is still in its infancy. As a result, not all doctors are equally informed and some of them accidentally prescribe the wrong vitamin D test. If you get the wrong test, you could test "normal" when you are anything but.

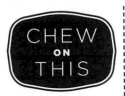
The D in a standard multivitamin and mineral supplement isn't enough D to get your levels up to normal. The amount of vitamin D in most vitamins is only 400 IU. It's not enough to prevent low blood levels or to bring low levels up to normal. Look for a stand-alone D supplement that contains 1,000 to 2,000 IU.

doctor's appointments, either. What to do? I recommend you do what The Endocrine Society recommends to keep blood levels above 30 ng/ml: Take a vitamin supplement. Unlike calcium, which often comes in a giant pill, D is small and easy to swallow. Use the following dosage guidelines:

YOU HAVE NO RISK FACTORS. Take 1,000 IU during the winter months.

YOU LIVE IN A NORTHERN CLIMATE, BUT ARE LIGHT SKINNED. Take 1,000 to 2,000 IU a day between November and March.

YOU LIVE IN A NORTHERN CLIMATE AND ARE RELIGIOUS ABOUT SUNSCREEN USE. Take 2,000 IU a day year-round.

YOU ARE A PERSON OF COLOR. Take 2,000 IU a day year-round, no matter where you live.

YOU ARE OVERWEIGHT OR OBESE. See a doctor. Physicians like Dr. Holick have superdosed their overweight and obese patients with D, trying to see just how much more supplemental D they needed in order to get their blood levels up to normal. As it turns out, it's double to triple what lean people need. I don't recommend you do this without the supervision of a doctor, though.

Only under the supervision of your doctor, Dr. Holick recommends 4,000 to 5,000 IU of D a day until your BMI drops below 30 and you are no longer considered obese by medical standards. He's done several studies that show that this amount is therapeutic, not toxic, even if administered for 6 months or longer.

Whatever supplement dose you take, combine it with the high-D menus in the coming chapters. A supplement alone will not slim you down. You need a supplement along with D-rich eating and portion control to drop pounds for good.

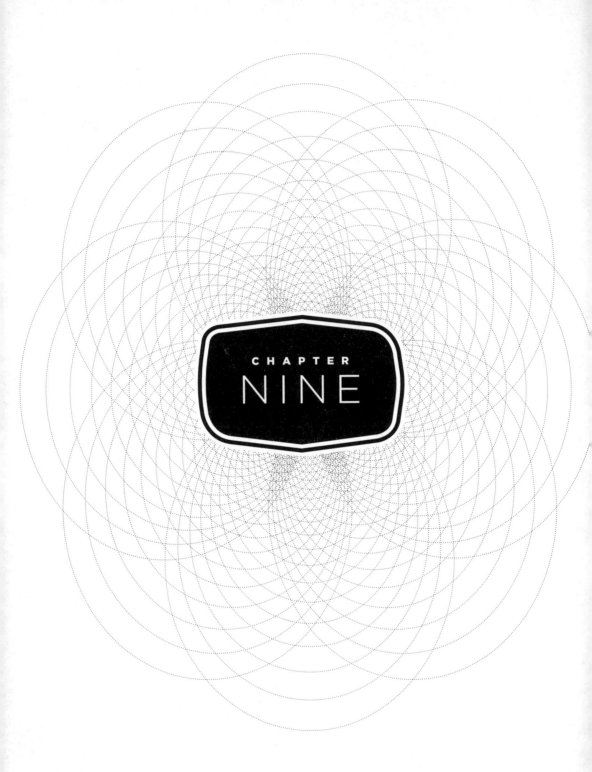

CHAPTER
NINE

The
7-Day
Slim
Down

In the following pages, you will find a week of menus that will superdose you with roughly 1,000 IU of vitamin D a day. Each day will also net you plenty of calcium and other nutrients that will work together synergistically to shift your body out of fat hoarding and into speed slimming. If you follow the plan as described, you will be well on your way to bringing your D stores back up to normal by week's end—and you can expect to drop up to 7 pounds. You'll also feel your energy levels increase, your mood lift, and maybe even your sex drive perk up. It's just the beginning of the new you!

Five Features of the Slim Down

1 **YOU'LL FOLLOW SET MENUS EACH DAY.** This is an important difference between The 7-Day Slim Down and The 4-Week Slim Down. In this first week of the program, I want to make sure you are providing your body with a steady dose of D throughout the day. I also want to make sure that your total dose of D by day's end tops the 1,000-IU mark. The only way to ensure you crest the 1,000-IU level is to design an entire day of eating for you.

2 **THESE MENUS ARE CALORIE CONTROLLED AT ROUGHLY 1,400 CALORIES A DAY.** As I've mentioned, optimizing D and other slimmers will help to speed your results, but portion control is still in order. Try to avoid extracurricular calorie consumption as much as possible. I've worked some beverages, such as orange juice and tea, into the plan. You may drink water, coffee, and tea (black, green, or herbal) throughout the day as needed. Minimize your consumption of carbonated beverages such as sodas, diet sodas, and sparkling water, as these tend to cause bloat and discomfort. Do not include extra beverage calories that are not included on the menus. Extra lattes, mixed drinks, or soda will provide you with extra calories that have not been accounted for on the plan, slowing or stalling your results.

3 **THE MENUS REPEAT.** You'll find three different daily menus that repeat once or twice throughout the week. I did this to save you money, time, and peace of mind. I know that it won't be easy to switch from your usual way of eating to slimmer eating. To help you make that transition, I've included several simple, quick-and-easy, or no-cook options. I've tried to keep the recipes you will use as minimal as possible, too. I've done all of this to reduce the number of new foods for you to shop for at the grocery store and the number of new recipes for you to familiarize yourself with in the kitchen. This way, you can shop once and use the same items over and over throughout the week. You can also make several meals in bulk, using the leftovers later in the week to save time. Another benefit is that you'll become more used to preparing these options, allowing them to become an automatic part of your dieting repertoire.

4 **I'VE PICKED YOUR SNACKS FOR YOU.** When you get to The 4-Week Slim Down, you'll be able to choose your snacks from a list of options. For this initial 7 days, however, the snacks are written into each day's choices. Again, I've done this to ensure you meet your total D goal for the day.

5 **YOU'LL DRINK GREEN TEA WITH MEALS AND SNACKS.** I've included green tea to help you speed your results even more. Note that green tea technology has dramatically improved in recent years. Many companies now make green tea that is mixed with other herbs like jasmine, cinnamon, or ginger, improving the taste. If you are starting this plan in the winter, you'll probably prefer hot green tea. If you are starting it in the summer, then definitely try the Bottomless Ginger Mint Iced (Green) Tea (page 210). This is a delicious tea mixture and will win you over, even if you think you hate the taste of green tea. Make a huge batch, keep it handy in your fridge, and drink it throughout the day or week.

Frequently Asked Questions

WHAT IF I DON'T LIKE THE MENU CHOICES ON A GIVEN DAY?
It's okay to swap one day for another. In fact, it's perfectly okay to repeat one day for the whole week, if that idea suits you. As long as each day's choices remain intact, you will be getting at least 1,000 IU of D by the day's end.

WHAT IF I CAN'T FIND SOMETHING ON A MENU? Just do the best you can. I've highlighted the D-rich foods. These are the most important ones to get right. Of those foods, only the mushrooms might be difficult for you to find. If you live in an area where D-rich mushrooms are not available, you have two options. You can take a vitamin D supplement to make up the difference (1,000 to 2,000 IU) or you can opt for menus that boost D with fish, eggs, and other options instead of mushrooms.

I'M A VEGETARIAN. WHAT SHOULD I DO? You can swap tofu for any source of meat you see on any given menu. Use the Swap This for That chart (page 166) for guidance.

I HATE GREEN TEA AND I'M NOT ABOUT TO CHANGE. WHAT SHOULD I DO? That's okay. Just swap coffee or some other calorie-free caffeine source for the tea. Or just drink water.

I ALWAYS HAVE A MORNING LATTE. CAN I STILL DO THIS ON THE PLAN? Yes, you can, but have it in place of one of the suggested snacks for the day. For instance, on day one, you can swap in your latte in place of the hard-cooked egg. Make sure you choose fat-free milk for your latte and do not include extras like sweeteners, which will add unnecessary calories. Also, hold yourself to a medium, rather than a large.

If you'd prefer to eat both of your snacks, here's another option: Go for regular drip coffee and use nondairy creamer in place of milk or cream.

I DON'T SEE ANY ALCOHOL LISTED ON THE SLIM DOWN. I LOVE A GLASS OF WINE WITH DINNER. CAN I STILL DO THAT? Ideally, you'll hold off on alcohol until you've finished the 7-Day Slim Down and are transitioning into the 4-Week Slim Down. Here's why: Alcohol lowers your inhibitions and intensifies cravings. That's the last thing you need during your first week of dieting.

That said, I'm all about options and freedom. If you absolutely feel you must have a nightly glass of wine, then count your alcoholic drink as one of your snacks for the day. For instance, on day one, you might substitute it for the cottage cheese with apple. Then make sure to hold yourself to just one 5-ounce glass, and don't overpour. In lieu of wine, you may also have one 12-ounce beer or the Orangetini (page 211).

How to Make the Most of the Slim Down

EAT AT HOME. Restaurant food generally contains an addictive combination of flavors (usually sweet plus salty) and ingredients that make it hard to stay in control (usually butter, salt, and sugar). It's also hard to ensure you are getting the right foods when you order. Most restaurants, for instance, do not use D-fortified products.

It's for this reason that I recommend you follow the Slim Down menus as prescribed and make your meals at home. Keep in mind that I am only suggesting you do this for 7 days and not for the rest of your life! Once you transition to the main plan, you can go back to eating at your favorite restaurants.

WRITE DOWN WHAT YOU EAT. Keeping a food diary is particularly helpful during the first week of the plan as you adjust to this new lifestyle. When you write down what you eat, it makes it a lot harder to overdo it on your portions and to indulge in extracurricular calories, explains Sari Greaves, RD, spokesperson for the American

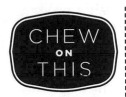

Seeing or smelling food can trigger a response in our brains that makes us feel hungry, even when we've just eaten. Override this response by serving your meal and then putting the rest away. If the rest of your family tends to eat seconds, then eat in a dining room but keep the serving bowls in the kitchen.

Dietetic Association. University of Pittsburgh researchers found that dieters who take note of what they eat lose weight more quickly than dieters who don't write it all down.

HIT THE REPLAY BUTTON. If you love a certain recipe, or even a whole day of meals, consider repeating it over and over and over again. The more often you make a recipe, the more it becomes ingrained and the easier it is for you to create. Repetition also helps you fill up on fewer calories, as research consistently shows that lots of variety in flavors and types of dishes tends to leave us feeling unsatisfied and craving more.

EAT ALL YOUR MEALS. Don't skip meals or skimp on portions in an attempt to lose weight more quickly. Those tactics will only backfire. Don't allow yourself to get overly hungry. It will reduce your resolve. Stick to the plan as written and you'll soon start to see results.

HEAT THINGS UP. Remember capsaicin, the optional fat burner I told you about earlier. Found in hot peppers, it has been shown to speed up your metabolism, so your body wastes calories as heat. That's why you feel hot and sweaty when you eat spicy food. Adding red pepper, jalapeños, or another hot spice to your meals will boost your weight loss. If you love spice, then use cayenne, jalapeños, and other hot spices liberally.

The Slim Down Shopping List

The following is a list of ingredients you'll need for this first week. If you are on a budget, note that it's perfectly okay to make substitutions.

PRODUCE

Apples, 2
Avocado, 1
Bananas
Bell peppers, 2
Berries, mixed, 1 cup
Broccoli florets, 2 cups
Brussels sprouts
Cantaloupe
Carrots
Cilantro, 1 bunch
Cucumbers, 3
Garlic
Ginger
Greens, mixed
Mushrooms, D-fortified,*
    3 packages
Onions, 5
Orange, 1
Potatoes, baking, 2
Scallions
Snow peas, 1 cup
Strawberries, 1 large
    package
Tomatoes, 2 large
Tomatoes, cherry,
    1 package

REFRIGERATED FOODS

Egg whites
Eggs, D-fortified*
Orange juice, D-fortified*

FROZEN FOODS

Frozen blackberries,
    strawberries,
    or raspberries
Frozen cauliflower

MEAT AND FISH

Chicken, sliced grilled,
    boneless, skinless
    breasts, 6 ounces each
Salmon, smoked, 8 ounces

Shrimp, medium, 4 ounces
Tilapia, 12 ounces
Tofu, Nasoya TofuPlus extra
    firm, 8 ounces
Turkey, fat-free, ground,
    2 pounds

DAIRY

Cheddar cheese, reduced-
    fat, shredded
Cheese, reduced-fat, sliced
Cottage cheese,* fat-free,
    medium container
Feta cheese, crumbed,
    1 small package
Milk, fat-free, D-fortified
Smart Balance Light
    Buttery Spread or any
    D-fortified soft tub trans
    fat–free margarine
Sour cream, reduced-fat,
    small container
Whipped topping, fat-free
Yogurt, D-fortified, fat-free,
    12 ounces
Yogurt, D-fortified, fat-free,
    vanilla 16 ounces

BREAD PRODUCTS

Thomas's Light Multi-Grain
    English Muffins
Whole grain bread,
    fortified*
Whole grain tortilla wraps,
    8 inches in diameter
Whole wheat
    hamburger buns

MISCELLANEOUS

Almonds, unsalted
Breakfast cereal,
    D-fortified*
Brown rice
Coffee, instant
Green tea

Pumpkin seeds
Walnuts
Wheat germ
Whole wheat penne, 1 box

CANNED AND JARRED FOODS

Artichoke hearts, 2 cans
Garbanzo beans, 1 can
Peppers, roasted, 1 jar
Pesto, reduced-fat
Salmon, wild, 3 cans
Salsa (optional)

PANTRY ITEMS AND SPICES

Cinnamon
Cocoa powder,
    unsweetened
Cornstarch
Crushed red pepper flakes
Garlic powder
Lemon juice
Lime juice
Mustard, dijon
Oil, canola
Oil, olive
Oil, sesame
Onion, minced, dried
Oregano, dried
Paprika
Parmesan cheese, grated
Parsley flakes, dried
Pepper, black
Romano cheese, grated
Salt
Soy sauce
Sugar
Vinegar, balsamic, and/or
    red wine vinegar
Worcestershire sauce

----

*See the Appendix (page 288)
    for recommended brands of
    D-fortified foods

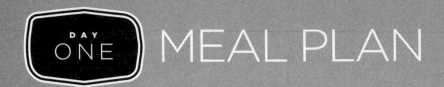

BREAKFAST

Cereal with Strawberries and Almonds

1 cup D-fortified cereal* (i.e., General Mills Total Wheat Flakes) with 1 cup D-fortified fat-free milk, 1 tablespoon chopped almonds, 1 cup strawberries, plus 4 ounces of calcium and D-fortified orange juice and green tea.

*Choose any cereal with 130 calories or less per 1-cup serving.

PER SERVING:
372 calories
283 IU vitamin D
1,946 mg calcium
18 g protein
72 g carbohydrates
4 g fat (<1 g saturated fat)
433 mg sodium
7 g fiber

MIDMORNING SNACK

▶ 1 D-fortified hard-cooked egg and green tea.

PER SERVING:
70 calories
80 IU vitamin D
26.5 mg calcium
6 g protein
<1 g carbohydrates
4 g fat (1.2 g saturated fat)
60 mg sodium
0 g fiber

LUNCH

Salmon over Mixed Greens

▶ 5 ounces of canned wild salmon, drained and mashed, on top of 2 cups mixed greens, 8 cherry tomatoes (halved), ½ sliced cucumber, 2 tablespoons garbanzo beans, 1 tablespoon crumbled feta cheese (optional), tossed with 1 teaspoon olive oil and 2 tablespoons balsamic vinegar (or red wine vinegar or 2 tablespoons reduced calorie dressing), with salt and pepper to taste.
▶ Green tea.

PER SERVING:
401 calories
660 IU vitamin D
521 mg calcium
40 g protein
28 g carbohydrates
14 g fat (3 g saturated fat)
993 mg sodium
6 g fiber

PER SERVING:
127 calories
0 IU vitamin D
65 mg calcium
14 g protein
17 g carbohydrates
1 g fat (<1 g saturated fat)
41 mg sodium
2 g fiber

MIDAFTERNOON SNACK

▶ ½ cup fat-free or 1% reduced-fat cottage cheese (optional: sprinkle with cinnamon) with ½ sliced apple and green tea.

PER SERVING:
492 calories
270 IU vitamin D
132 mg calcium
30 g protein
56 g carbohydrates
17 g fat (3 g saturated fat)
282 mg sodium
11 g fiber

DINNER

Penne with Mushrooms and Artichokes with Salad

▶ 1 serving Penne with Mushrooms and Artichokes (page 224) tossed with 2 ounces sliced, grilled, boneless, skinless chicken breast (optional). Serve with salad of leafy greens, sliced tomato, cucumber, 1 tablespoon chopped walnuts, with 1 tablespoon olive oil and balsamic vinegar.

Total Day One

1,463 CALORIES, **1,293** IU VITAMIN D, **2,691** MG CALCIUM, **108** G PROTEIN, **174** G CARBOHYDRATES, **41** G FAT (8.2 G SATURATED FAT), **1,810** MG SODIUM, **26** G FIBER.

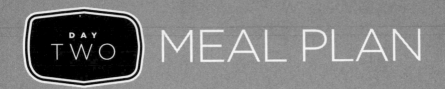

BREAKFAST

Lox, Eggs, and Onions

▸ 1 serving Lox, Eggs, and Onions (page 215) with
1 slice D-fortified whole wheat (or whole grain) toast*
and 1 teaspoon Smart Balance Light Buttery Spread or any
D-fortified soft tub trans fat–free margarine, 1 cup cantaloupe and 4 ounces D-fortified orange juice and green tea

*Choose any D-fortified, reduced-calorie whole grain or whole wheat
bread with 80 calories or less per slice.*

PER SERVING:
333 calories
424 IU vitamin D
368 mg calcium
18 g protein
43 g carbohydrates
10 g fat (3 g saturated fat)
448 mg sodium
4 g fiber

MIDMORNING SNACK

▸ ½ banana with 2 tablespoons reduced-fat sour cream and
green tea.

PER SERVING:
107 calories
3 IU vitamin D
45 mg calcium
3 g protein
16 g carbohydrates
4 g fat (3 g saturated fat)
22 mg sodium
2 g fiber

LUNCH

Turkey Mushroom Burger with Sliced Peppers and Cucumber

▸ 1 serving of Turkey Mushroom Burgers (page 216) on
a D-fortified whole wheat hamburger bun* (optional) and
1 ounce reduced-fat cheese (optional) plus 1 cup raw sliced
peppers and 1 sliced cucumber drizzled with ½ teaspoon
olive oil, 1 or 2 tablespoons red wine vinegar or fresh lemon
juice, pinch of salt, and pepper and dried oregano to taste.

Choose any D-fortified hamburger bun with 120 calories or less.

PER SERVING:
452 calories
324 IU vitamin D
366 mg calcium
43 g protein
43 g carbohydrates
12 g fat (2 g saturated fat)
817 mg sodium
8 g fiber

PER SERVING:
131 calories
91 IU vitamin D
285 mg calcium
9 g protein
18 g carbohydrates
3 g fat (<1 g saturated fat)
64 mg sodium
2 g fiber

MIDAFTERNOON SNACK

▶ 1 serving Chocolate Mocha Smoothie (page 211)

PER SERVING:
366 calories
279 IU vitamin D
132 mg calcium
42 g protein
28 g carbohydrates
11 g fat (3 g saturated fat)
610 mg sodium
6 g fiber

DINNER

Parmesan Tilapia with Brussels Sprouts and Baked Potato

▶ Preheat the oven to 350°F. Season 6 ounces tilapia with dried minced onion, dried parsley flakes, paprika, garlic powder, black pepper, and crushed red pepper flakes (optional). Top with 1 tablespoon of grated Parmesan cheese and 1 teaspoon Smart Balance Light Buttery Spread or any D-fortified soft tub trans fat–free margarine. Bake for 8 to 10 minutes or until fish is opaque. Serve with 1 cup brussels sprouts roasted with 1 teaspoon olive oil and salt and pepper to taste; and $\frac{1}{2}$ plain baked potato (optional: add 1 tablespoon salsa).

Total Day Two

1,389 CALORIES, **1,120** IU VITAMIN D, **1,195** MG CALCIUM,

115 G PROTEIN, **148** G CARBOHYDRATES, **39** G FAT (11 G SATURATED FAT),

1,961 MG SODIUM, **20** G FIBER.

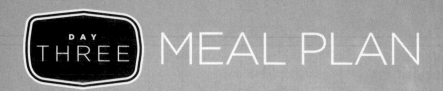
BREAKFAST

Berry Yogurt with Scrambled Eggs

▶ 6 ounces D-fortified fat-free yogurt with ½ cup mixed berries topped with 1 tablespoon wheat germ plus 1 D-fortified egg and 2 egg whites scrambled in a nonstick pan, salt and pepper to taste. Serve with 1 slice D-fortified whole wheat (or whole grain) bread and 1 teaspoon D-fortified soft tub trans fat–free margarine (optional).

PER SERVING:
347 calories
257 IU vitamin D
464 mg calcium
27 g protein
41 g carbohydrates
8 g fat (2 g saturated fat)
708 mg sodium
4 g fiber

MIDMORNING SNACK

▶ 10 unsalted almonds plus 4 ounces calcium and D-fortified orange juice and green tea.

PER SERVING:
131 calories
50 IU vitamin D
209 mg calcium
4 g protein
16 g carbohydrates
7 g fat (<1 g saturated fat)
<1 mg sodium
1 g fiber

LUNCH

Mushroom Onion Avocado Quesadilla and Salad

▶ Sauté 2 ounces D-fortified sliced mushrooms and ¼ cup chopped onion in 1 teaspoon oil until browned. Combine ¼ avocado and 1 teaspoon chopped cilantro and spread on ½ 8″ soft tortilla wrap. Top with 4 tablespoons reduced-fat shredded Cheddar cheese and mushroom onion mixture, fold in half, and cook in a heated nonstick pan 3 to 4 minutes per side or until lightly browned. Serve with leafy greens, tomato, cucumber, 1 teaspoon toasted pumpkin seeds, 1 teaspoon olive oil, and lemon juice, salt and pepper to taste.

PER SERVING:
386 calories
267 IU vitamin D
348 mg calcium
15 g protein
30 g carbohydrates
25 g fat (7 g saturated fat)
404 mg sodium
6 g fiber

PER SERVING:
164 calories
103 IU vitamin D
413 mg calcium
11 g protein
27 g carbohydrates
2 g fat (1 g saturated fat)
171 mg sodium
2 g fiber

MIDAFTERNOON SNACK

▶ 1 serving Fruit Smoothie (page 212)

PER SERVING:
448 calories
268 IU vitamin D
150 mg calcium
17 g protein
69 g carbohydrates
12 g fat (1 g saturated fat)
878 mg sodium
11 g fiber

DINNER

Seared Shrimp with Stir–Fried Vegetables and Brown Rice

▶ 1 serving Seared Shrimp with Stir-Fried Vegetables (page 240) plus ¾ cup cooked brown rice and 1 orange, sliced.

Total Day Three

1,487 CALORIES, **944 IU VITAMIN D,** **1,585** MG CALCIUM,

74 G PROTEIN, **183** G CARBOHYDRATES, **53** G FAT (12 G SATURATED FAT),

2,162 MG SODIUM, **24** G FIBER.

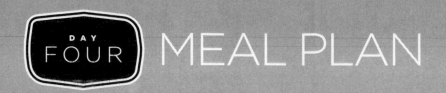
BREAKFAST

Cereal with Strawberries and Almonds

▸ 1 cup D-fortified cereal* (i.e., General Mills Total Wheat Flakes) with 1 cup D-fortified fat-free milk, 1 tablespoon chopped almonds, 1 cup strawberries plus 4 ounces calcium and D-fortified orange juice and green tea.

Choose any cereal with 130 calories or less per 1-cup serving

PER SERVING:
372 calories
283 IU vitamin D
1,946 mg calcium
18 g protein
72 g carbohydrates
4 g fat (<1 g saturated fat)
433 mg sodium
7 g fiber

MIDMORNING SNACK

▸ 1 D-fortified hard-cooked egg and green tea

PER SERVING:
70 calories
80 IU vitamin D
27 mg calcium
6 g protein
<1 g carbohydrates
4 g fat (1 g saturated fat)
60 mg sodium
0 g fiber

LUNCH

Salmon over Mixed Greens

▸ 5 ounces canned wild salmon, drained and mashed, on top of 2 cups mixed greens, 8 cherry tomatoes (halved), ½ sliced cucumber, 2 tablespoons garbanzo beans, 1 tablespoon crumbled feta cheese (optional) tossed with 1 teaspoon olive oil and 2 tablespoons balsamic vinegar (or red wine vinegar or 2 tablespoons reduced-calorie dressing), and salt and pepper to taste.
▸ Green tea.

PER SERVING:
401 calories
660 IU vitamin D
521 mg calcium
40 g protein
28 g carbohydrates
14 g fat (3 g saturated fat)
993 mg sodium
6 g fiber

MIDAFTERNOON SNACK

▸ ½ cup fat-free or 1% reduced-fat cottage cheese (optional: sprinkle with cinnamon) with ½ sliced apple and green tea.

DINNER

Penne with Mushrooms and Artichokes with Salad

▸ 1 serving Penne with Mushrooms and Artichokes (page 224) tossed with 2 ounces sliced, grilled, boneless, skinless chicken breast (optional) plus salad of leafy greens, sliced tomato, cucumber, 1 tablespoon chopped walnuts with 1 tablespoon olive oil and balsamic vinegar.

Total Day Four

1,463 CALORIES, **1,293** IU VITAMIN D, **2,691** MG CALCIUM, **108** G PROTEIN, **174** G CARBOHYDRATES, **41** G FAT (11 G SATURATED FAT), **1,810** MG SODIUM, **26** G FIBER.

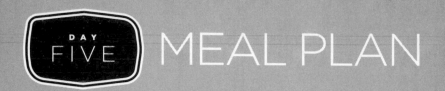

BREAKFAST

Lox, Eggs, and Onions

▶ 1 serving Lox, Eggs, and Onions (page 215) with
1 slice D-fortified whole wheat (or whole grain) toast*
and 1 teaspoon Smart Balance Light Buttery Spread or any
D-fortified soft tub trans fat–free margarine, 1 cup cantaloupe, and 4 ounces D-fortified orange juice and green tea

*Choose any D-fortified reduced-calorie whole grain or whole wheat
bread with 80 calories or less per slice.*

PER SERVING:
333 calories
424 IU vitamin D
368 mg calcium
18 g protein
43 g carbohydrates
10 g fat (3 g saturated fat)
448 mg sodium
4 g fiber

MIDMORNING SNACK

▶ ½ banana with 2 tablespoons reduced-fat sour cream and
green tea

PER SERVING:
107 calories
3 IU vitamin D
45 mg calcium
3 g protein
16 g carbohydrates
4 g fat (3 g saturated fat)
22 mg sodium
2 g fiber

LUNCH

Turkey Mushroom Burger with Sliced Peppers and Cucumber

▶ 1 serving of Turkey Mushroom Burgers (page 216) on
a D-fortified whole wheat hamburger bun* (optional) and
1 ounce reduced-fat cheese (optional) plus 1 cup raw sliced
peppers and 1 sliced cucumber drizzled with ½ teaspoon
olive oil, 1 or 2 tablespoons red wine vinegar or fresh lemon
juice, pinch of salt, and pepper and dried oregano to taste.

Choose any D-fortified hamburger bun with 120 calories or less.

PER SERVING:
452 calories
324 IU vitamin D
366 mg calcium
43 g protein
43 g carbohydrates
12 g fat (2 g saturated fat)
817 mg sodium
8 g fiber

PER SERVING:
131 calories
91 IU vitamin D
285 mg calcium
9 g protein
18 g carbohydrates
3 g fat (<1 g saturated fat)
64 mg sodium
2 g fiber

MIDAFTERNOON SNACK

▶ 1 serving Chocolate Mocha Smoothie (page 211)

PER SERVING:
366 calories
279 IU vitamin D
132 mg calcium
42 g protein
28 g carbohydrates
11 g fat (3 g saturated fat)
610 mg sodium
6 g fiber

DINNER

Parmesan Tilapia with Brussels Sprouts and Baked Potato

▶ Preheat the oven to 350°F. Season 6 ounces tilapia with dried minced onion, dried parsley flakes, paprika, garlic powder, black pepper, and crushed red pepper flakes (optional). Top with 1 tablespoon of grated Parmesan cheese and 1 teaspoon Smart Balance Light Buttery Spread or any D-fortified soft tub trans fat–free margarine. Bake for 8 to 10 minutes or until fish is opaque. Serve with 1 cup brussels sprouts roasted with 1 teaspoon olive oil and salt and pepper to taste; and 1/2 plain baked potato (optional: add 1 tablespoon salsa).

Total Day Five

1,389 CALORIES, **1,120** IU VITAMIN D, **1,195** MG CALCIUM,

115 G PROTEIN, **148** G CARBOHYDRATES, **39** G FAT (11 G SATURATED FAT),

1,961 MG SODIUM, **20** G FIBER.

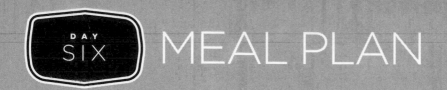

BREAKFAST

Berry Yogurt with Scrambled Eggs

▶ 6 ounces D-fortified fat-free yogurt with ½ cup mixed berries topped with 1 tablespoon wheat germ plus 1 D-fortified egg and 2 egg whites scrambled in a nonstick pan, salt and pepper to taste. Serve with 1 slice D-fortified whole wheat (or whole grain) bread and 1 teaspoon D-fortified soft tub trans fat-free margarine (optional).

PER SERVING:
347 calories
257 IU vitamin D
464 mg calcium
27 g protein
41 g carbohydrates
8 g fat (2 g saturated fat)
708 mg sodium
4 g fiber

MIDMORNING SNACK

▶ 10 unsalted almonds plus 4 ounces calcium and D-fortified orange juice and green tea.

PER SERVING:
131 calories
50 IU vitamin D
209 mg calcium
4 g protein
16 g carbohydrates
7 g fat (<1 g saturated fat)
<1 mg sodium
1 g fiber

LUNCH

Mushroom Onion Avocado Quesadilla and Salad

▶ Sauté 2 ounces D-fortified sliced mushrooms and ¼ cup chopped onion in 1 teaspoon oil until browned. Combine ¼ avocado and 1 teaspoon chopped cilantro and spread on ½ 8″ soft tortilla wrap. Top with 4 tablespoons reduced-fat shredded Cheddar cheese and mushroom onion mixture, fold in half, and cook in a heated nonstick pan 3 to 4 minutes per side or until lightly browned. Serve with leafy greens, tomato, cucumber, 1 teaspoon toasted pumpkin seeds, 1 teaspoon olive oil, lemon juice, and salt and pepper to taste.

PER SERVING:
386 calories
267 IU vitamin D
348 mg calcium
15 g protein
30 g carbohydrates
25 g fat (7 g saturated fat)
404 mg sodium
6 g fiber

PER SERVING:
164 calories
103 IU vitamin D
413 mg calcium
11 g protein
27 g carbohydrates
2 g fat (1 g saturated fat)
171 mg sodium
2 g fiber

MIDAFTERNOON SNACK

▶ 1 serving Fruit Smoothie (page 212)

PER SERVING:
448 calories
268 IU vitamin D
150 mg calcium
17 g protein
69 g carbohydrates
12 g fat (1 g saturated fat)
878 mg sodium
11 g fiber

DINNER

Seared Shrimp with Stir–Fried Vegetables and Brown Rice

▶ 1 serving Seared Shrimp with Stir-Fried Vegetables (page 240) plus ¾ cup cooked brown rice and 1 orange, sliced.

Total Day Six

1,478 CALORIES, **944** IU VITAMIN D, **1,585** MG CALCIUM,
74 G PROTEIN, **183** G CARBOHYDRATES, **53** G FAT (12 G SATURATED FAT),
2,162 MG SODIUM, **24** G FIBER.

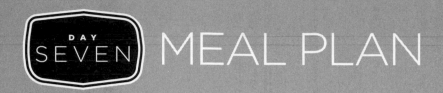

MEAL PLAN

BREAKFAST

Cereal with Strawberries and Almonds

▶ 1 cup D-fortified cereal* (i.e., General Mills Total Wheat Flakes) with 1 cup D-fortified fat-free milk, 1 tablespoon chopped almonds, 1 cup strawberries plus 4 ounces calcium and D-fortified orange juice and green tea.

Choose any cereal with 130 calories or less per 1-cup serving

PER SERVING:
372 calories
283 IU vitamin D
1,946 mg calcium
18 g protein
72 g carbohydrates
4 g fat (<1 g saturated fat)
433 mg sodium
7 g fiber

MIDMORNING SNACK

▶ 1 D-fortified hard-cooked egg and green tea.

PER SERVING:
70 calories
80 IU vitamin D
27 mg calcium
6 g protein
<1 g carbohydrates
4 g fat (1 g saturated fat)
60 mg sodium
0 g fiber

LUNCH

Salmon over Mixed Greens

▶ 5 ounces canned wild salmon, drained and mashed, on top of 2 cups mixed greens, 8 cherry tomatoes (halved), ½ sliced cucumber, 2 tablespoons garbanzo beans, 1 tablespoon crumbled feta cheese (optional) tossed with 1 teaspoon olive oil and 2 tablespoons balsamic vinegar (or red wine vinegar or 2 tablespoons reduced-calorie dressing), and salt and pepper to taste.
▶ Green tea.

PER SERVING:
401 calories
660 IU vitamin D
521 mg calcium
40 g protein
28 g carbohydrates
14 g fat (3 g saturated fat)
993 mg sodium
6 g fiber

PER SERVING:
127 calories
0 IU vitamin D
65 mg calcium
14 g protein
17 g carbohydrates
1 g fat (<1 g saturated fat)
41 mg sodium
2 g fiber

MIDAFTERNOON SNACK

▶ ½ cup fat-free or 1% reduced-fat cottage cheese
(optional: sprinkle with cinnamon) with ½ sliced apple
and green tea.

PER SERVING:
492 calories
270 IU vitamin D
132 mg calcium
30 g protein
56 g carbohydrates
17 g fat (3 g saturated fat)
282 mg sodium
11 g fiber

DINNER

Penne with Mushrooms and Artichokes with Salad

▶ 1 serving Penne with Mushrooms and Artichokes (page
224) tossed with 2 ounces sliced, grilled, boneless, skinless
chicken breast (optional) plus salad of leafy greens, sliced
tomato, cucumber, 1 tablespoon chopped walnuts with
1 tablespoon olive oil and balsamic vinegar.

Total Day Seven

1,463 CALORIES, **1,293** IU VITAMIN D, **2,691** MG CALCIUM,
108 G PROTEIN, **174** G CARBOHYDRATES, **41** G FAT (8 G SATURATED FAT),
1,810 MG SODIUM, **26** G FIBER.

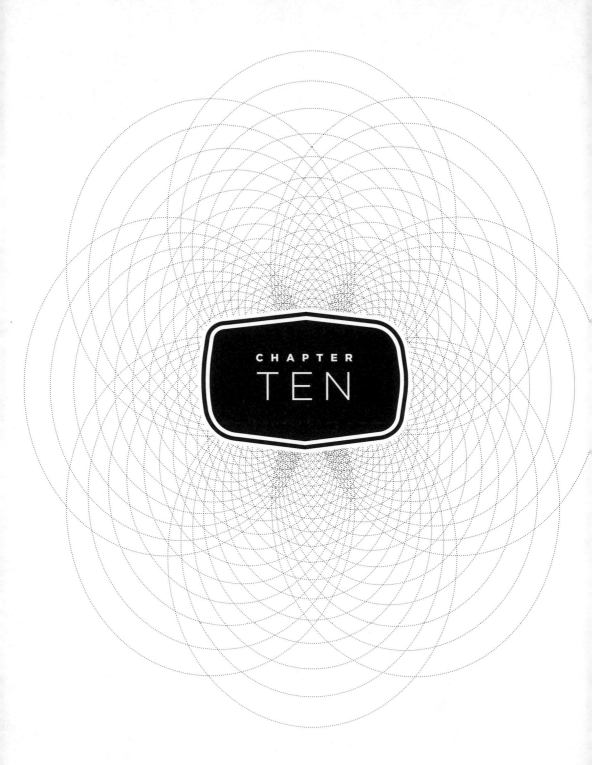

CHAPTER
TEN

The 4-Week Slim Down

Are you ready to discover a brand-new you? You are about to embark on a supercharged plan that maximizes several fat-burning nutrients—especially vitamin D—to help you drop pounds in record time and reveal your slimmest, sexiest self!

In the following pages, you'll find 4 weeks' worth of menu options for breakfast, lunch, dinner, and snacks. Like the 7-Day Slim Down, these options are designed to superdose your body with D in order to get stores up to normal.

Unlike the Slim Down, however, you will now be in the driver's seat. This is important because you need flexibility in order to stay true to any diet. You might be able to follow a strict day-by-day plan for 7 days, but 4 weeks and beyond is another story. That's why in the following pages you'll find dozens of mix-and-match options for breakfast, lunch, dinner, and snacks. Use these options to design a winning menu plan that suits your taste buds, lifestyle, and budget.

Five Features of the Slim Down

1 **THERE ARE NO SET DAILY MENUS.** Create a personalized, winning menu based on the options provided. This plan lets you pick what works best for you and omit what doesn't. Every single option listed in the following pages contains a hefty dose of both vitamin D and calcium. No matter what options you choose, you will be superdosing your body with powerful fat melters. By the end of each day, the menu options will have provided you with a minimum of 400 IU of D and 1,000 milligrams of calcium no matter which ones you try. In reality, you'll probably net closer to 600 IU, and some days you'll even crest 1,000 IU.

2 **THIS PLAN WORKS IN CONJUNCTION WITH THE WINTER AND SUMMER MENUS.** Think of The 4-Week Slim Down as your main plan and the winter menus (Chapter 11) and summer menus (Chapter 12) as auxiliary plans that you will add and drop depending on the time of year. You'll use The 4-Week Slim Down no matter what time of year you start the diet. But if you are starting this plan during the winter, then I highly encourage you to incorporate the winter options in Chapter 11 right away as they will boost your D even more, as well as help satisfy any yearnings you might have for warming foods. If you are starting the plan in the summer, definitely incorporate summer options, too.

3 **YOU GET TO PICK YOUR OWN SNACKS.** Use the list that is provided.

4 **YOU WON'T SEE GREEN TEA LISTED WITH EACH MEAL.** That doesn't mean you should drop it. If you don't mind drinking green tea, then keep up the habit. It will continue to speed your results.

5 **NOW IS THE TIME FOR DRINKING AND EATING OUT.** Just be mindful of the rules of success that we've already discussed, especially the 90/10 principle. When you indulge consciously, you'll be more likely to satisfy cravings and stick to your diet.

How to Follow the Slim Down

THE SLIM DOWN is designed around 4 weeks of customizable menus, but it's also designed to teach you new eating habits to help you reach your goals and maintain them for a lifetime.

For optimal success, remember the following:

Eat the options you want when you want. All of the options are interchangeable. You can eat breakfast for dinner, lunch for breakfast, or make any other switch you can think of.

Stick to the suggested portions. The menu options are all calorie and portion controlled. It's important to make and consume the correct portions. Little cheats like adding another slice of cheese or extra salad dressing can add up and slow your results.

Purchase the right foods. Not all foods are created equal when it comes to vitamin D. Make sure to read the "Pick This, Not That" section carefully and consult the list of recommended brands in the Appendix (page 288).

Choose the right snacks. Choose from among the recommended snacks on pages 170 to 171. Just remember: Indulge only twice per day. You can have a glass of wine when you're out with friends on Saturday night, or a special latte on a Saturday morning. And you can have dessert after dinner, too. But you can't do all of it on the same Saturday. You can have up to two snacks a day on this plan, so I recommend you make one healthy. Then make the other whatever you want, as long as it is only 100 calories.

Watch those liquid calories. Whether it's soda, juice, or wine, keep in mind that all of these liquids have a caloric cost. Nothing is off-limits on this plan, but all of it must be accounted for if you want to consistently lose weight. Count liquid calories as one of your snacks, and make sure these drinks don't go over your calorie budget. Each of your two daily snacks is designed to total no more than 100 calories. A small nonfat cappuccino will be just about right, but a large mocha will put you way over your limit.

Automate your eating. Don't feel guilty about picking the same favorites day after day. This can actually help you shed fat faster by reducing stress. As I've mentioned, it's difficult to learn how to shop for, store, and prepare lots of new recipes and menus. If you opt for a few favorites over and over again, you'll be able to do a lot of this prep work without doing much extra work. You'll know what to buy without using a list, and you'll know how to prepare it, too.

Look for my great eat-out options. I've marked several options in this plan as easily found in restaurants. (Look for this info next to the individual recipe titles.) In some cases you'll want to make a substitution or two, and I've provided that information for you as well.

How to Follow the Slim Down at Restaurants

USE THE LIST of recommended restaurant options in the Appendix for guidance for eating out. In addition, follow this advice:

STICK TO A CALORIE BUDGET. Dinners should total about 400 calories. If you'd like to eat a bit more, combine your meal with your snack, so you have a total of 500 calories to work with. And as a general rule of thumb, eat only half of whatever you are served, as many restaurants serve super-sized portions that can add up to more than 1,000 calories. (Ask to box up the remaining portion and bring it home for a convenient leftover meal to eat another time.)

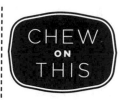

CHEW
ON
THIS

More restaurants are supplying calorie details, but some restaurants only offer calorie info for certain items. Why? In general, restaurants only provide calorie info for low-calorie items and not high-calorie items. So if an item does not have calorie info, you can bet that it totals 1,000 calories or more! This is even true of salads.

USE THE D-SMART FORMULA. Try to find entrées that include a high-D food, a high-calcium food, and some vegetables, for example, wild salmon on salad greens with a little cheese.

SWAP LOW-D CHOICES FOR HIGHER-D ONES WHENEVER POS-SIBLE. Ask for fish instead of chicken, oysters instead of clams, and milk instead of alcohol or a soft drink.

CHOOSE LEAN CUTS OF MEAT OVER FATTIER OPTIONS. Ask for poultry or soy instead of red meat (especially for burgers) and skinless options. This helps you cut calories, which is important when you're eating out. Restaurant food is often loaded with fat and calories, so you need to make a greater effort at portion and calorie control than you would at home.

Lose Weight During the Holidays

SOMETIMES YOU JUST want to indulge—holidays and celebrations are usually those times. It's really okay, every once in a while, to take a break from this plan. For instance, let's say that it's Thanksgiving, and you just want to eat everything that's on the table—and nothing on the table resembles anything that is recommended on this plan.

Here's what to do: Combine lunch with dinner on that big day. Eat in the middle of the afternoon or a little later. Try to eat no more than 800 calories for your meal. If you can swing some healthy choices in that meal (whole grains, vegetables, fruit, lean protein), great. If not, at least abide by the 800-calorie limit, using a calorie counter for guidance.

Then, the very next day, get right back on track, picking up on the diet where you left off.

Supercharge Your Results

THE 4-WEEK SLIM DOWN is already front-loaded with nutrients that will help you shed fat fast. Still, you can speed your results even more by optimizing D and aiming for 1,000 IU a day rather than just 600. To do that, you'll want to pick one "Supercharged" menu option marked with an asterisk. This will put you over the 1,000-IU level for the day so you can rebuild your D stores quickly and keep your fat-burners on high.

To get a sense of what this looks like, look at the menu makeovers below. Keep in mind that you probably don't need or want to eat supercharged menus every single day. But it's a good idea to have these foods in mind when you feel you need to ramp up your menus and keep those fires burning.

Menu Makeovers

	BREAKFAST	LUNCH	DINNER	TOTAL
NOT SUPER-CHARGED!	Almond Butter Toast with Yogurt and Granola Crunch (121 D)	Creamy Banana Smoothie with Fruit (182)	Chicken in a Skillet with Cous Cous (186)	**489 IU** vitamin D
SUPER-CHARGED!	Lox, Eggs, and Onion with Toast and Cantaloupe (382)	Mushroom, Onion, and Avocado Quesadilla Salad (267)	Halibut with Brown Rice, Mushroom Pilaf, and Swiss Chard (602)	**1,251 IU** vitamin D
SUPER-CHARGED!	Scrambled Eggs in a Pita (351)	Caesar Salad with Salmon and Toasted Parmesan Pita (660)	Chicken Cacciatore with Sautéed Escarole (272)	**1,283 IU** vitamin D
SUPER-CHARGED!	Cereal with Strawberries and Almonds (283)	Portobello Sandwich with Coleslaw (403)	Salmon with Millet Salad and Snow Peas (625)	**1,311 IU** vitamin D

Cheat and Still Slim Down

THERE ARE GOING to be times in your life when you just can't stick to these menu options: during the holidays, when you're traveling, and, occasionally, when you're in a rut and craving something different. Remember the 90/10 principle! If you stick to the plan 90 percent of the time, you'll be in great shape and continue to see success. The other 10 percent of the time, keep this advice in mind.

→ **Always control your portions.** If you're eating out, ask for calorie information. Keep your meals to 400 calories or fewer. When in doubt, eat only half of what you are served. Use the eating out guide in the Appendix for help.

→ **Boost your supplement.** It's a good idea to double up on your D supplement during extended periods of travel and during other periods of time when you can't follow the menus as easily. Rather than taking only 1,000 IU daily, increase your dosage to 2,000 IU until you can follow the menus again.

→ **Make smart swaps.** There will be times when you just can't bring yourself to consume another bite of fish, another egg, or some other high-D food. That's okay. Use the chart below to make smart substitutions for any of the menu options.

SWAP THIS	FOR THAT
5 ounces sirloin, flank steak, tenderloin, ham, Canadian bacon, pork tenderloin, skinless chicken, or venison	5 ounces salmon, halibut, or any other fish
4 ounces tofu	1 ounce any other lean meat or fish
Any nonstarchy, low-calorie vegetable (broccoli, bell pepper, spinach, cucumbers, etc.)	Sliced mushrooms or any other vegetable on the plan

The Slimming Sandwich

IN ADDITION TO the times you'll want to "cheat," there will also be times when you're just in a rush and need something fast. That's where sandwiches come in! They're easy, portable, and fit into any setting. You can bring a sandwich to work or a picnic and no one will suspect you are on a diet. Use this formula to make your own high-D sandwiches.

CHOOSE ONE OF EACH:

Bread	Protein	Produce	Toppings
Choose a brand with no more than 150 calories per serving.	*Choose one. Bolded items are preferred because they are high in D and/or calcium.*	*Choose an unlimited amount of any of these.*	*Choose one.*
1 or 2 slices D-fortified, reduced-calorie bread (for a total of 150 calories)	**1 cooked egg + 1 slice low-fat cheese**	Lettuce Alfalfa sprouts Sliced bell pepper	1 Tbsp reduced-calorie mayo One 50-calorie serving of your favorite sand-wich spread
1 D-fortified English muffin	**2 cooked eggs** **4–5 oz sliced tofu, grilled or baked**	Sliced cucumber Sliced onion	¼ avocado, mashed or sliced
1 whole grain wrap (about 6–8" in diameter)	**4 oz canned salmon or tuna (packed in water)**	Sliced tomato	2 Tbsp mustard
1 whole grain pita	3–4 ounces lean lunch meat (turkey, roast beef, or ham) 3 ounces sliced low-fat cheese		1 tsp pesto 2 Tbsps hummus

The Slim Down Pantry List

BECAUSE YOU'LL be mixing and matching the options on pages 172 through 185 based on your tastes and lifestyle, I can't provide you with a definitive shopping list. What follows, however, are pantry items that you'll want to keep on hand, along with a few fresh foods that you will probably use quite often.

FREQUENTLY USED FRESH FOODS

Bananas
Berries (strawberries, blueberries)
Chicken breast, fresh skinless
Eggs, omega-3
Grapefruit
Greens, leafy salad
Margarine, high-D
Milk, fat-free, D-fortified
Mushrooms, D-fortified
Orange juice, D-fortified
Salmon, wild, fresh
Tofu, D-fortified, extra-firm
Whole grain bread, D-fortified
Whole grain burger buns
Whole grain English muffins
Whole grain pitas
Yogurt, fat-free, D-fortified

PANTRY STAPLES

Artichokes, canned
Beans, canned (chickpeas, black, kidney)
Cereal, breakfast, D-fortified
Cereal, low-fat granola, D-fortified
Nut butters, unsalted (peanut, almond, etc.)
Nuts and seeds (walnuts, almonds, and others)
Salmon, wild, canned
Sardines, canned
Tea, green
Tuna, canned, packed in water

FREEZER STAPLES

Frozen fruit
Whole grain frozen waffles

Pick This, Not That

YOU'LL FIND A detailed list of recommended brands in the Appendix. That list will take some of the label reading out of your grocery shopping exercise as I've done the research for you. That said, more and more D-fortified foods are hitting the market every day, so keep an eye out for great new choices like the ones I list here!

PICK THIS	NOT THAT
Dried shiitake mushrooms	Fresh low-D shiitake mushrooms
Omega-3 eggs (such as Eggland's Best brand)	Regular eggs
Wild salmon	Farm-raised salmon
Canned tuna	Tuna steak
Mushrooms with vitamin D (such as Monterey Mushrooms brand)	Regular mushrooms
D-fortified yogurt and kefir	Regular yogurt and kefir
D-fortified OJ	Regular OJ
D- and calcium-fortified tofu	Regular tofu

Your Supercharged Snack List

CHOOSE UP TO TWO SNACKS a day from this list. Super-charged snacks are in bold. I've included calorie counts for your convenience. But as long as you're choosing two of these recommended snacks per day, there's no need to count calories!

1 D-fortified hard-cooked egg (Eggland's Best - 70 calories)

½ cup fat-free or 1% reduced-fat cottage cheese with ½ sliced apple (127 calories)

½ banana with 2 tablespoons reduced-fat sour cream (107 calories)

10 unsalted almonds plus 4 ounces calcium- and D-fortified orange juice (131 calories)

1 tablespoon reduced-fat peanut butter + ½ sliced apple (140 calories)

2 teaspoons reduced-fat peanut butter + 1 apple (157 calories)

1 rice cake, lightly salted, with 1 tablespoon peanut butter (129 calories)

3 tablespoons hummus plus 1 whole sliced and peeled cucumber (109 calories) or 5 medium celery stalks (107 calories)

3 tablespoons guacamole plus 1 whole sliced and peeled cucumber (102 calories) or 5 medium celery stalks (100 calories)

1 serving Chocolate Mocha Smoothie (page 212, 131 calories)

1 serving Fruit smoothie (page 212, 164 calories)

½ serving Green tea and blueberry smoothie (page 213, 93 calories)

½ serving of Kefir Banana Froth (page 213, 113 calories)

½ serving Creamy Banana Breakfast Smoothie (page 228, 157 calories)

½ serving Pineapple Mango Smoothie (page 214, 119 calories)

½ serving Almond Smoothie (page 214, 126 calories)

6 ounces fat-free flavored yogurt (80–100 calories)

½ cup 1% reduced-fat cottage cheese mixed with cinnamon or nutmeg (80 calories)

1 fat-free string cheese stick or 1 ounce fat-free or low-fat cheese (80 calories)

20 whole strawberries (80 calories)

1 cup blueberries (83 calories)

1 cup raspberries (64 calories)

1 cup blackberries (62 calories)

2 plums (60 calories)

1 mango or papaya (125–130 calories)

1 pear (96 calories)

1 apple (94 calories)

4 or 5 dates (90–120 calories)

1 cup unsweetened applesauce (100 calories)

1 large orange (62 calories)

1 large peach (60 calories)

1 medium banana (100 calories)

½ cantaloupe (94 calories)

½ cantaloupe with ¼ cup cottage cheese, nonfat or 1% (134 calories)

1½ cups honeydew melon (96 calories)

2 cups watermelon (91 calories)

1 cup grapes (104 calories)

1 whole grapefruit (103 calories)

½ cup edamame (boiled soybeans, lightly salted and shelled) (100 calories)

10 unsalted almonds (77 calories) or 10 unsalted raw cashews (½ ounce, 81 calories)

2 tablespoons dry-roasted sunflower seeds (93 calories)

2 tablespoons pistachio nuts (87 calories)

4 cups yellow air-popped popcorn (124 calories) or 3 cups white air-popped popcorn (122 calories)

12 ounces fat-free cappuccino (Starbucks, 60 calories)

16 ounces fat-free cappuccino (Starbucks, 80 calories)

12 ounces 2% cappuccino (Starbucks, 90 calories)

16 ounces 2% cappuccino (Starbucks, 120 calories)

12 ounces soy milk cappuccino (Starbucks, 80 calories)

16 ounces soy milk cappuccino (Starbucks, 110 calories)

12 ounces fat-free caffè latte (Starbucks, 100 calories)

16 ounces fat-free caffè latte (Starbucks, 130 calories)

12 ounces 2% caffè latte (Starbucks, 150 calories)

12 ounces soy milk caffè latte (Starbucks, 130 calories)

12 ounces fat-free caffè misto (Starbucks, 60 calories)

16 ounces fat-free caffè misto (Starbucks, 70 calories)

12 ounces 2% caffè misto (Starbucks, 80 calories)

16 ounces 2% caffè misto (Starbucks, 110 calories)

12 ounces soy milk caffè misto (Starbucks, 70 calories)

16 ounces soy milk caffè misto (Starbucks, 100 calories)

1 Hazelnut Latte (page 211, 134 calories)

1 Orangetini (page 211, 152 calories)

5-ounce glass red or white wine (120–130 calories)

3-ounces sake (117 calories)

12 ounces regular beer (+/-150 calories)

12 ounces light beer (+/-100 calories)

12 ounces nonalcoholic beer (65 calories)

½ cup Jell-O instant pudding mix (sugar-free, reduced-calorie) prepared with D-fortified fat-free milk (70–80 calories)

Swiss Miss Great Start Cocoa (110 calories)

VitaTops Apple Crumb muffin (100 calories)

One 100-calorie serving of your favorite dark chocolate

2 dark chocolate Dove bar miniatures (84 calories)

2 Hershey Special Dark miniatures (80 calories)

2 squares Ghirardelli dark chocolate (10 calories)

Breakfast Options

Banana–Nut Hot Cereal

▶ 1 packet D-fortified Instant Hot Cereal (Cream of Wheat Healthy Grain Instant—Original) with ¾ cup D-fortified fat-free milk, 2 teaspoons chopped walnuts, and ½ sliced banana, sprinkled with cinnamon or nutmeg (optional).

Eat-Out Tip: If you can't find fortified Cream of Wheat, oatmeal will work in a pinch. If the restaurant makes the hot cereal with water instead of milk, ask for the milk on the side, mixing some of it into your cereal and drinking the rest. It's okay to go without the nuts and spices if the restaurant doesn't serve them. It's also okay to swap the banana for half of another type of fruit, such as half of an apple or orange.

PER SERVING:
317 calories
175 IU vitamin D
506 mg calcium
17 g protein
57 g carbohydrates
4 g fat (<1 g saturated fat)
298 mg sodium
8 g fiber

Cereal with Strawberries and Almonds

▶ 1 cup D-fortified cereal* (such as General Mills Total Wheat Flakes) with 1 cup D-fortified fat-free milk, 1 tablespoon chopped almonds, and 1 cup strawberries, plus 4 ounces of calcium- and D-fortified orange juice.

Choose any cereal with 130 calories or less per 1-cup serving.

Eat-Out Tip: If the restaurant doesn't have almonds, go ahead and skip them. If the restaurant doesn't have strawberries, you can substitute half a piece of another type of fruit, such as half an apple or banana.

PER SERVING:
372 calories
283 IU vitamin D
1,946 mg calcium
18 g protein
72 g carbohydrates
4 g fat (<1 g saturated fat)
433 mg sodium
7 g fiber

PER SERVING:
404 calories
130 IU vitamin D
603 mg calcium
14 g protein
69 g carbohydrates
9 g fat (2 g saturated fat)
542 mg sodium
7 g fiber

Waffles, Yogurt and Sparkling OJ

▸ 2 frozen whole wheat (or multigrain) waffles topped with 6 ounces D-fortified fat-free yogurt,* 1 tablespoon ground flaxseed, and 1/2 cup blueberries, plus 4 ounces calcium- and D-fortified orange juice combined with 4 ounces sparkling sodium-free club soda (optional).

Choose any plain or flavored yogurt with 100 calories or less per 6-ounce serving.

PER SERVING:
378 calories
121 IU vitamin D
513 mg calcium
16 g protein
57 g carbohydrates
11 g fat (1 g saturated fat)
251 mg sodium
6 g fiber

Almond Butter Toast with Yogurt and Granola Crunch

▸ 6 ounces D-fortified fat-free yogurt* with 2 tablespoons low-fat granola cereal; 1/2 grapefruit; and 1 slice D-fortified whole grain (whole wheat) bread** with 1 tablespoon unsalted almond butter (or any unsalted nut butter).

Choose any plain or flavored yogurt with 100 calories or less per 6-ounce serving.

**Choose any D-fortified reduced-calorie whole grain or whole wheat bread with 80 calories or less per slice.*

PER SERVING:
347 calories
257 IU vitamin D
464 mg calcium
27 g protein
41 g carbohydrates
8 g fat (2 g saturated fat)
708 mg sodium
4 g fiber

Berry Yogurt with Scrambled Eggs

▸ 6 ounces D-fortified fat-free yogurt* with 1/2 cup mixed berries topped with 1 tablespoon wheat germ plus 1 D-fortified egg and 2 egg whites scrambled in a nonstick pan, with salt and pepper to taste. Serve with 1 slice D-fortified whole wheat (or whole grain) bread and 1 teaspoon Smart Balance Light Buttery Spread or any D-fortified soft tub trans fat–free margarine (optional).

Choose any plain or flavored yogurt with 100 calories or less per 6-ounce serving.

Creamy Banana Smoothie with Fruit

▶ 1 serving Creamy Banana Breakfast Smoothie (page 228) with 1 cup mixed berries (or 1 orange, ½ cup mango, or ½ grapefruit).

PER SERVING:
378 calories
182 IU vitamin D
589 mg calcium
20 g protein
67 g carbohydrates
5 g fat (<1 g saturated fat)
130 mg sodium
7 g fiber

Hard-Cooked Eggs with Turkey Bacon and Smoothie

▶ 2 D-fortified hard-cooked eggs with 2 slices low-sodium turkey bacon and 1 serving Green Tea and Blueberry Smoothie (page 213).

PER SERVING:
376 calories
217 IU vitamin D
215 mg calcium
20 g protein
43 g carbohydrates
13 g fat (4 g saturated fat)
341 mg sodium
4 g fiber

Lox, Eggs, and Onions with Toast and Cantaloupe

▶ 1 serving Lox, Eggs, and Onions (page 215) with 1 slice D-fortified whole wheat toast* and 1 teaspoon Smart Balance Light Buttery Spread or any D-fortified soft tub trans fat-free margarine and 1 cup cantaloupe.

Choose any D-fortified reduced-calorie whole grain or whole wheat bread with 80 calories or less per slice.

PER SERVING:
278 calories
374 IU vitamin D
193 mg calcium
17 g protein
31 g carbohydrates
10 g fat (3 g saturated fat)
448 mg sodium
4 g fiber

Scrambled Eggs in a Pita

PER SERVING:
351 calories
345 IU vitamin D
266 mg calcium
26 g protein
34 g carbohydrates
15 g fat (4 g saturated fat)
766 mg sodium
11 g fiber

▸ Coat a skillet with nonstick cooking spray and add 1 teaspoon olive or canola oil. Sauté 1 tablespoon chopped onion, 6 cherry tomatoes (halved), 1 cup baby spinach leaves, ½ cup D-fortified sliced mushrooms, and salt and pepper to taste. Remove from pan when soft. Scramble 2 D-fortified eggs with 2 tablespoons D-fortified fat-free milk and 1 tablespoon reduced-fat Cheddar cheese. Combine eggs and vegetables in 1 whole wheat pita.*

Choose any whole-wheat pita with 100 calories or less.

Asparagus Mushroom and Mozzarella Omelet

Great Eat-Out Option!

PER SERVING:
371 calories
260 IU vitamin D
483 mg calcium
30 g protein
23 g carbohydrates
17 g fat (8 g saturated fat)
834 mg sodium
3 g fiber

▸ Coat a skillet with nonstick cooking spray and add 1 teaspoon olive or canola oil. Sauté ½ cup D-fortified mushrooms and ¼ cup chopped asparagus until soft. Add salt and pepper to taste. Pour 1 D-fortified egg with 2 egg whites (beaten) into pan and let set, add 2 ounces part-skim mozzarella cheese and cook until firm. Fold over and serve with 1 cup mixed fruit salad.

Eat-Out Tip: Substitute whatever vegetable the restaurant offers in place of the asparagus, such as green peppers, mushrooms, or broccoli. Most restaurants will mix the whole eggs with the egg whites upon request. Ask them to go "light on the cheese" since the cheese will probably be full-fat.

Lunch and Dinner Options

ALL LUNCH AND dinner options are interchangeable. Remember to choose D-fortified products over their regular counterparts.

Steak with Portobello Barley and Broccoli

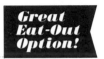

Great Eat-Out Option!

▶ 5 ounces broiled lean steak (trimmed of all fat) plus
1 serving of Portobello Mushroom Barley (page 226) and
1 cup steamed broccoli.

Eat-Out Tip: If the restaurant doesn't serve barley, opt for the
same amount of another grain, preferably a whole grain like brown
rice if you can find it.

PER SERVING:
414 calories
142 IU vitamin D
80 mg calcium
39 g protein
26 g carbohydrates
17 g fat (6 g saturated fat)
261 mg sodium
7 g fiber

Turkey Mushroom Burger with Sliced Peppers and Cucumber

▶ 1 serving of Turkey Mushroom Burgers (page 216) on
1 D-fortified whole wheat hamburger bun* (optional) with
1 ounce reduced-fat cheese (optional), plus 1 cup raw sliced
peppers and 1 sliced cucumber drizzled with ½ teaspoon
olive oil, 1 or 2 tablespoons red wine vinegar or fresh lemon
juice, pinch of salt, and pepper and dried oregano to taste.

Choose any D-fortified hamburger bun with 120 calories or less.

PER SERVING:
452 calories
324 IU vitamin D
366 mg calcium
43 g protein
43 g carbohydrates
12 g fat (2 g saturated fat)
817 mg sodium
8 g fiber

Spicy Meatballs in Marinara Sauce with Whole Wheat Pasta and Mixed Greens

PER SERVING:

503 calories
280 IU vitamin D
422 mg calcium
24 g protein
70 g carbohydrates
14 g fat (2 g saturated fat)
1,296 mg sodium
9 g fiber

▶ 1 serving Spicy Meatballs in Marinara Sauce (page 217) plus unlimited mixed leafy greens tossed with 2 tablespoons reduced-calorie balsamic vinaigrette dressing.

Chicken Cacciatore with Sautéed Escarole

PER SERVING:

386 calories
272 IU vitamin D
110 mg calcium
33 g protein
37 g carbohydrates
13 g fat (2 g saturated fat)
670 mg sodium
8 g fiber

▶ 1 serving Chicken Cacciatore (page 218) plus 1½ cups chopped escarole leaves sautéed in 1 teaspoon olive oil, with sliced garlic clove, salt and pepper to taste, and sprinkled with crushed red pepper flakes (optional).

Chicken in a Skillet with Couscous

PER SERVING:

371 calories
186 IU vitamin D
201 mg calcium
46 g protein
26 g carbohydrates
8 g fat (3 g saturated fat)
568 mg sodium
3 g fiber

▶ 1 serving Chicken in a Skillet (page 219) plus ½ cup cooked plain couscous mixed with ½ teaspoon chopped almonds and 1 teaspoon chopped parsley.

Salmon Burger Salad with Corn on the Cob

▸ 1 Salmon Burger (see page 220) with sliced tomato on top of 2 cups mixed field greens and 1 medium ear of corn with 1 teaspoon Smart Balance Light Buttery Spread or any D-fortified soft tub trans fat–free margarine (optional).

PER SERVING:
431 calories
476 IU vitamin D
407 mg calcium
32 g protein
60 g carbohydrates
9 g fat (2 g saturated fat)
647 mg sodium
9 g fiber

Salmon with Millet Salad and Snow Peas

▸ 5 ounces of grilled, baked, or broiled wild pacific salmon at desired temperature coated with 1 tablespoon of low-sodium soy sauce and served with 1/2 cup cooked millet* mixed with 1 teaspoon chopped scallions, 1 teaspoon olive oil, 1 or 2 tablespoons balsamic vinegar, and 1/2 cup steamed snow peas

You can substitute amaranth or quinoa for the millet.

PER SERVING:
457 calories
625 IU vitamin D
76 mg calcium
38 g protein
41 g carbohydrates
14 g fat (2 g saturated fat)
771 mg sodium
4 g fiber

Caesar Salad with Grilled Salmon and Toasted Parmesan Pita (OPTION A)

Great Eat-Out Option!

▸ 5 ounces grilled, baked, or broiled wild pacific salmon (with 1 teaspoon olive oil and salt and pepper to taste) at desired temperature over 2 cups romaine lettuce and 2 tablespoons reduced-calorie Caesar dressing (i.e., Newman's Own Lighten Up Salad Caesar Dressing) plus 1 whole wheat pita* brushed with 1 teaspoon olive oil and sprinkled with 1 teaspoon grated Parmesan cheese, then toasted.

Choose any whole wheat pita with 100 calories or less.

PER SERVING:
474 calories
625 IU vitamin D
165 mg calcium
40 g protein
30 g carbohydrates
25 g fat (4 g saturated fat)
1,017 mg sodium
11 g fiber

Caesar Salad with Salmon and Toasted Parmesan Pita (OPTION B)

▶ 5 ounces canned wild salmon with bones (drained and mashed) over 2 cups romaine lettuce and 2 tablespoons of reduced-calorie Caesar dressing (i.e., Newman's Own Lighten Up Salad Caesar Dressing) plus 1 whole wheat pita* brushed with 1 teaspoon olive oil and sprinkled with 1 teaspoon grated Parmesan cheese, then toasted.

Choose any whole wheat pita with 100 calories or less.

Tuna Melt and Salad

▶ 4 ounces light tuna packed in water, drained and mixed with 1 chopped scallion. In a separate bowl, combine 1 tablespoon olive oil, 1½ tablespoons balsamic vinegar, and a pinch of ground black pepper. Set aside 1 tablespoon of the mixture, then add 1 tablespoon D-fortified fat-free plain yogurt. Stir in tuna and scallions. Spread onto 1 slice D-fortified whole wheat or whole grain bread* and top with 1 slice reduced-fat cheese. Broil until browned. Serve with 1 cup mixed lettuce, ½ cup chopped red pepper, and 1 tablespoon of reserved dressing mixture.

Choose any D-fortified reduced-calorie whole grain or whole wheat bread with 80 calories or less per slice.

Eat-Out Tip: The restaurant will probably serve you too much tuna made with full-fat mayo. Make sure to compensate by eating only a half portion.

Spicy Tuna in a Pita with Carrots, Tomatoes, and Avocado

▶ 4 ounces of light tuna packed in water, drained, mixed with 2 tablespoons mild, medium, or hot salsa, 2 table- spoons chopped red onion, 2 teaspoons reduced-fat mayonnaise, 1 teaspoon Dijon mustard, Tabasco sauce, salt and pepper to taste. Stuff into ½ whole wheat pita* with shredded lettuce. Serve with 1 cup baby carrots, 1 cup cherry tomatoes, and ½ sliced avocado.

Choose any whole wheat pita with 100 calories or less.

PER SERVING:
435 calories
205 IU vitamin D
155 mg calcium
40 g protein
48 g carbohydrates
13 g fat (2 g saturated fat)
1,273 mg sodium
19 g fiber

||||||||||||||||||||||||||||||||||||||||||||||||||||||||||||||||||||||||||||||||||||||||||||||||||||||||||||

Tuna Tacos with Sliced Peppers and Guacamole

Great Eat-Out Option!

▶ 1 serving Tuna Tacos (page 221) with 1 cup sliced peppers and ¼ cup guacamole. (Optional: Add Tabasco sauce.)

Eat-Out Tip: This is a great Tex-Mex option. You can substitute whatever type of fish comes in the fish tacos the restaurant prepares. Make sure to watch your guacamole portion, as the restaurant will probably serve you way too much.

PER SERVING:
455 calories
259 IU vitamin D
80 mg calcium
32 g protein
33 g carbohydrates
23 g fat (5 g saturated fat)
457 mg sodium
10 g fiber

||||||||||||||||||||||||||||||||||||||||||||||||||||||||||||||||||||||||||||||||||||||||||||||||||||||||||||

Puttanesca Pizza with Mixed Green Salad

▶ 1 serving Puttanesca Pizza (page 222) with (1½) cups mixed greens, (5) cherry tomatoes (halved), (½) cup sliced cucumber, ¼ cup chopped artichoke hearts, 2 tablespoons garbanzo beans, 1 tablespoon olive oil, and 2 tablespoons balsamic vinegar or lemon juice.

Note: Salad amounts are in () since calories are negligible and can be unlimited unless specified.

PER SERVING:
372 calories
242 IU vitamin D
248 mg calcium
31 g protein
43 g carbohydrates
10 g fat (3 g saturated fat)
661 mg sodium
9 g fiber

PER SERVING:
412 calories
471 IU vitamin D
119 mg calcium
32 g protein
32 g carbohydrates
10 g fat (3 g saturated fat)
548 mg sodium
8 g fiber

Baked Halibut with Sweet Potato

▶ Marinate 5 ounces halibut in 1 tablespoon lemon juice, ⅛ teaspoon salt, and ¼ teaspoon paprika in a shallow baking dish coated with nonfat cooking spray. Cover and refrigerate for 1 hour. Sauté ½ cup red bell pepper and ½ cup sliced onion in 1 tablespoon Smart Balance Light Buttery Spread or any D-fortified soft tub trans fat–free margarine in a nonstick skillet. Preheat the oven to 450°F. Top the halibut with the peppers and onions and bake for 10 minutes or until opaque. Serve with 1 medium baked sweet potato and 1 tablespoon reduced-fat sour cream (optional).

PER SERVING:
513 calories
602 IU vitamin D
168 mg calcium
38 g protein
50 g carbohydrates
19 g fat (3 g saturated fat)
842 mg sodium
8 g fiber

Halibut with Brown Rice Mush-room Pilaf and Swiss Chard

▶ Preheat the oven to 450°F. Bake 5 ounces halibut topped with mixture of 2 tablespoons seasoned breadcrumbs and 1 teaspoon olive oil for 10 minutes or until opaque. Serve with 1 serving Brown Rice Mushroom Pilaf (page 227) and 1 cup steamed Swiss chard.

PER SERVING:
409 calories
156 IU vitamin D
260 mg calcium
22 g protein
67 g carbohydrates
7 g fat (<1 g saturated fat)
811 mg sodium
16 g fiber

Miso Glazed Shrimp with Brown Rice and Bok Choy

▶ 1 serving Miso Glazed Shrimp and Shiitake Mushrooms (page 223) with ¾ cup cooked brown rice and 1 cup bok choy, sautéed in 1 teaspoon canola oil.

Parmesan Tilapia with Brussels Sprouts and Baked Potato

▶ Preheat the oven to 350°F. Season 6 ounces tilapia with dried minced onion, dried parsley flakes, paprika, garlic powder, black pepper, and crushed red pepper flakes (optional) and top with 1 tablespoon grated Parmesan cheese and 1 teaspoon Smart Balance Light Buttery Spread (or any D-fortified soft tub trans fat–free margarine). Bake for 8 to 10 minutes or until fish is opaque. Serve with 1 cup brussels sprouts roasted with 1 teaspoon olive oil and salt and pepper to taste and ½ plain baked potato (optional: add 1 tablespoon salsa).

PER SERVING:
366 calories
279 IU vitamin D
132 mg calcium
42 g protein
28 g carbohydrates
11 g fat (3 g saturated fat)
610 mg sodium
6 g fiber

Tilapia with Black Beans, Kale, and Quinoa

▶ Sauté 2 tablespoons chopped onion seasoned with fennel seeds and salt to taste in 2 teaspoons olive oil until onions are soft. Add 1 cup chopped kale leaves to skillet. When kale begins to wilt, stir in ¼ cup black beans (rinsed and drained), add 5 ounces tilapia to the pan, dust with paprika, and cover until fish is cooked through. Serve with ½ cup cooked quinoa.

PER SERVING:
452 calories
210 IU vitamin D
164 mg calcium
44 g protein
38 g carbohydrates
15 g fat (2 g saturated fat)
326 mg sodium
9 g fiber

Sardine and Egg Sandwich

▶ Drain 1 can sardines in oil. Place sardines on whole wheat roll* with 1 sliced D-fortified hard-cooked egg, sliced red onion, romaine lettuce, and tomato. Spread with 1 teaspoon reduced-fat mayonnaise and 1 teaspoon Dijon mustard. Serve with raw celery and carrots.

Choose any whole wheat roll with 130 calories or less.

PER SERVING:
457 calories
258 IU vitamin D
436 mg calcium
37 g protein
38 g carbohydrates
17 g fat (3 g saturated fat)
965 mg sodium
8 g fiber

Penne with Mushrooms and Artichokes and Green Salad

▸ 1 serving Penne with Mushrooms and Artichokes (page 224). Toss in 2 ounces sliced, grilled, boneless, skinless chicken breast (optional). Serve with salad of leafy greens, sliced tomato, and cucumber, tossed with 1 tablespoon olive oil, 2 tablespoons balsamic vinegar, and salt and pepper to taste.

Eat-Out Tip: If you cannot find a pasta combo like the one suggested here, ask for plain pasta or another grain on the side.

Szechuan Eggplant and Tofu with Brown Rice and Broccoli

▸ 1 serving Szechuan Eggplant and Tofu (page 225) plus ½ cup cooked brown rice and 1 cup steamed broccoli.

Portobello Sandwich with Coleslaw

▸ Top 3-ounce, grilled D-fortified whole portobello mushroom with sautéed ¼ cup sliced onion and ¼ cup bell pepper (in 1 teaspoon olive oil), then cover 1 slice reduced-fat cheese and bake for 5 minutes. Place on 2 toasted slices D-fortified whole wheat (or whole grain) bread with 1 teaspoon prepared pesto (optional). Serve with 2 cups shredded coleslaw mix tossed with 2 table-spoons reduced-calorie dressing (i.e., Newman's Own Lighten Up Dressing)

Mushroom Onion Avocado Quesadilla and Salad

▶ Sauté 2 ounces D-fortified sliced mushrooms and ¼ cup chopped onion in 1 teaspoon oil until browned. Combine ½ avocado and 1 teaspoon chopped cilantro and spread on ¼ 8" soft tortilla wrap. Top with 4 tablespoons reduced-fat shredded Cheddar cheese and mushroom-onion mixture, fold in half, and cook in a heated nonstick pan 3 to 4 minutes per side or until lightly browned. Serve with leafy greens, tomato, cucumber, 1 teaspoon toasted pumpkin seeds, 1 teaspoon olive oil, lemon juice, and salt and pepper to taste.

PER SERVING:
386 calories
267 IU vitamin D
348 mg calcium
15 g protein
30 g carbohydrates
25 g fat (7 g saturated fat)
404 mg sodium
6 g fiber

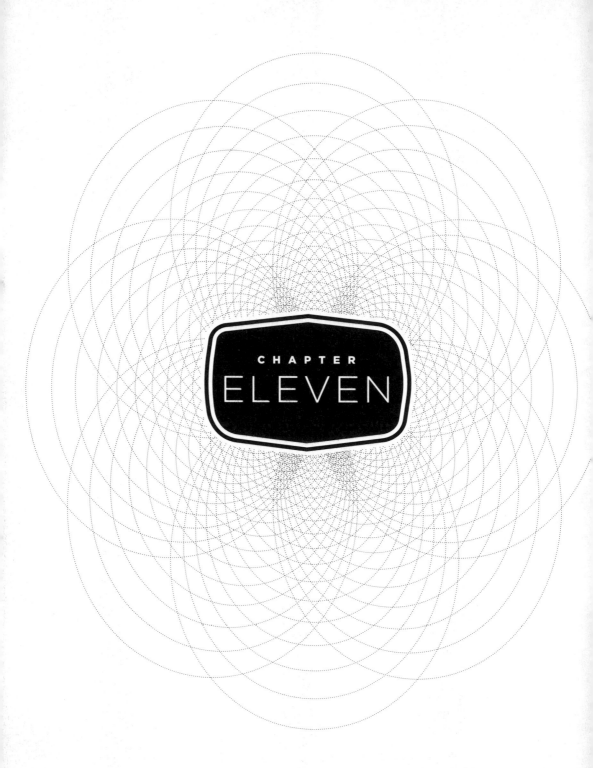

CHAPTER

ELEVEN

Winter Warming Menus

I n the following pages, you'll find 10 menu suggestions for the cold, dark winter months. Consume these meals as needed when the days are short and the nights are long. They will help to boost mood, reduce cravings, and warm you up during the winter months. Use them as an adjunct to the 4-week menu options, mixing them into your weekly repertoire as needed.

Four Features of the Winter Warming Plan

1 **ALL OF THESE MEALS CONTAIN UP TO DOUBLE THE D.** It's much more important to optimize D during the winter months, especially if you live north of Atlanta. During these months of the year, there just isn't enough sunlight for you to keep your D stores up to normal. As the days grow short, your body will steal D from various tissues and you will eventually become suboptimal or deficient. That's why these menus are all superdosed with D. Some provide more than 1,000 IU per meal, whereas the lowest D suggestions still offer a good 300 IU.

2 **THESE MEALS WILL STICK TO YOUR RIBS.** I don't know about you, but two of the last things I ever want to eat during the long winter months are salads and smoothies. Yet most diets absolutely require you to subsist on such foods no matter the time of year. This is not one of those diets. Your winter menu is loaded with the very foods you will crave during the winter months. The following 10 recipes and meals (pages 193 to 195) are all hearty, warming meals. We're talking soups, stews, and heavier, satisfying flavors.

3 **THERE ARE BIGGER PORTIONS FOR BIGGER APPETITES.** These meals are heartier than many of the 4-week options.

They will help you to feel more satisfied during the months when you are usually the most tempted to overeat.

4 YOU CAN TRANSITION TO WINTER EATING SEAMLESSLY.
That's because these menu options work in conjunction with The 4-Week Slim Down. You can mix and match them with the list of menu suggestions you already have.

How to Follow the Winter Menus

THE WINTER MENUS are designed to help you get suboptimal levels of D up to normal during the winter months, when you can't rely on sunlight for help. For best results, follow these pointers:

➜ **COMBINE THIS PLAN WITH A SUPPLEMENT.** Everyone, no matter their skin type, should be taking a 1,000 to 2,000 IU vitamin D supplement between the months of November and March. If you are a person of color, opt for the higher dose. If you are light skinned, you might be able to get away with the lower dose.

➜ **FOLLOW THE SAME RULES YOU DID FOR THE SLIM DOWN.** As with the 4-week plan, portion control is still important. The menu options are all calorie and portion controlled. It's important to make and consume the correct portions. Little cheats can add up and slow your results. Also, remember to purchase the right foods. Don't forget to choose from among the recommended brands in the Appendix and to follow the advice in the "Pick This, Not That" on page 169.

➜ **STICK WITH THE FOODS YOU LOVE.** If you love the 4-week plan and it's working for you, you do not have to work in the winter options. They are here for you when you need them, but they are not required.

Supercharge Your Results Even More

TWO THINGS HAPPEN during the winter months that make it harder to stick to your diet. The first is that it gets cold! You're more likely to be bundled up in lots of layers and wanting to cuddle up with a hot bowl of macaroni and cheese than you are to be picnicking outdoors with a fresh salad. The second is that the darker days trigger seasonal depression, which can lead to cravings and an effort to comfort yourself by giving in to those cravings. These cravings can be for crunchy and salty, sweet and creamy, or a combination.

The winter menu will help to prevent the winter munchies because you will be dosing yourself with enough D to bolster your mood and reduce cravings. Here's some additional advice to stoke those fat-burning fires and keep you on track.

➜ **Use warming herbs.** Certain types of herbs can really warm you up. They include: ginger, cayenne, cardamom, cinnamon, and garlic. To make a really super warming ginger tea, use fresh gingerroot, found in most supermarkets. Grate it and simmer in hot water for 5 to 10 minutes before straining. You can also use herbal tea bags. As I've already mentioned, cayenne not only warms you up, it also speeds your metabolism. Add a sprinkle of hot red pepper to any dish to boost your results and keep cravings under wraps.

➜ **Opt for snacks that satisfy.** Don't make the mistake of eating around a craving. If you need some crunch, then have it. If you need a little sweet and creamy, find the right snack, and enjoy the recommended portion. The worst thing you can do is eat and eat and eat so-called healthy foods—and still go over your calorie limit. Whenever possible, try to stop winter cravings by having a cup of warm tea before indulging.

➜ **Stay warm.** Invest in silk underwear or a cashmere wrap. The more you can stay warm and comfortable, the less likely you are to reach for food that will mimic this feeling of comfort. Treat yourself to a nonfood reward for sticking to your plan, like shearling-lined slippers—a toasty reminder of your progress!

The Winter Soup Maker

SOUP IS A STAPLE in my home in the winter. Once a week, I love to make a huge pot of it that I store and dip into for the rest of the week. There's just something about it that satisfies every part of my being. It smells lovely, which lifts my mood. It's also warm. And it's high in volume, but low in calories—which helps to turn down that vicious winter appetite. Various studies done at Penn State have shown that soup is a wonderful addition to a weight-loss menu. When dieters consume it regularly, they lose weight because it fills them up on fewer calories.

You'll find several soup and stew recipes and menus in the following pages. To create your own soups, use the following formula: Start your soup by sautéing any onions, garlic, and root vegetables in a little oil. Then add your liquid base and build the soup from there. Cook any pasta or starchy vegetables separately and add them to your soup just before serving. This will ensure they remain al dente and do not overcook. You can purchase stock or make your own.

THE WARMING SOUP FORMULA
This formula yields one large serving of soup for one person. Each serving equals 400 calories. Double, triple, or quadruple the amounts to yield as many servings as you'd like to prepare.

CHOOSE FROM EACH ROW:

LIQUID BASE *1–2 cups water + one of the following*	• 1 cup reduced-sodium vegetable stock • 1 cup reduced-sodium chicken stock	• 1 cup reduced-sodium beef stock • 1 cup fish stock	
VEGGIES *(Pick two)*	• 1 cup mushrooms • Onion, to taste • Garlic, to taste • 1 cup diced carrots	• 1 cup diced celery • 1½ cups chopped kale	• 3 cups chopped spinach • 1½ cups green beans
PROTEIN *Match your protein to your liquid base. (Pick one)*	• 3 ounces wild salmon • 4 ounces shrimp	• 4 ounces boneless skinless chicken breast	• 3 ounces extra-lean ground beef or ground poultry
FILLINGS *(Pick one)*	• ¾ cup diced potatoes • ½ cup cooked pasta • ½ cup cooked beans (white, red, black, garbanzo, etc.)	• ¾ cup corn off the cob • ¾ cup sweet potato or yam, cubed • 1½ cups winter squash	• ½ cup cooked barley • ½ cup cooked lentils
HERBS, SPICES, AND FLAVOR- INGS *Use any herb or spice, to taste + one of the following (optional):*	• 1 Tbsp reduced-fat sour cream (add at end after removing soup from heat and allowing to cool for 4–5 minutes)	• 1 Tbsp reduced-fat cream cheese (add at end after removing soup from heat and allowing to cool for 4–5 minutes)	• 1 Tbsp tomato puree • 2 tsp pesto

Winter Menu Plan

Add these savory meals during the winter months to boost your Vitamin D intake.

PER SERVING:
500 calories
638 IU vitamin D
253 mg calcium
43 g protein
60 g carbohydrates
12 g fat (4 g saturated fat)
626 mg sodium
12 g fiber

Wild Mushroom and Beef Stew with Wild Rice and Carrots

▸ 1 serving Wild Mushroom and Beef Stew (page 229) with ½ cup cooked wild rice and 1 cup steamed carrots

PER SERVING:
488 calories
338 IU vitamin D
74 mg calcium
35 g protein
57 g carbohydrates
16 g fat (4 g saturated fat)
857 mg sodium
10 g fiber

Beef Barley Soup and Whole Grain Crackers

▸ 1 serving Beef Barley Soup (page 228) with 120 calories' worth of whole grain crackers (i.e., 1 serving Kashi Heart to Heart Original Crackers)

PER SERVING:
418 calories
789 IU vitamin D
49 mg calcium
31 g protein
28 g carbohydrates
19 g fat (4 g saturated fat)
753 mg sodium
12 g fiber

Chicken Scallopini with Garlic Mushroom Sauce and Artichoke

▸ 1 serving Chicken Scallopini with Garlic Mushroom Sauce (page 230) plus 1 large steamed artichoke with 2 tablespoons melted Smart Balance Light Buttery Spread or any D-fortified soft tub trans fat–free margarine mixed with lemon juice and zest, for dipping

Sesame Crusted Salmon with Green Beans and Tomato Salad

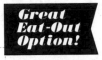

▶ 1 serving Sesame Crusted Salmon (page 231) plus ½ sliced or chopped tomato drizzled with 1 teaspoon olive oil, 1 tablespoon balsamic vinegar, salt, pepper to taste, and topped with 1 tablespoon chopped basil

Eat-Out Tip: Swap a basic green salad (no cheese, no croutons) for the tomato salad if tomato salad isn't on the menu.

PER SERVING:
475 calories
628 IU vitamin D
126 mg calcium
38 g protein
19 g carbohydrates
28 g fat (6 g saturated fat)
421 mg sodium
6 g fiber

Orange Poached Salmon with Star Anise, Spinach, and Roasted Cauliflower

▶ 1 serving Orange Poached Salmon with Star Anise and spinach (page 232) plus 1 cup roasted cauliflower

PER SERVING:
396 calories
800 IU vitamin D
266 mg calcium
41 g protein
25 g carbohydrates
15 g fat (2 g saturated fat)
244 mg sodium
4 g fiber

Catfish Fingers with Spicy Mayonnaise and Sweet Potato

▶ 1 serving Catfish Fingers with Spicy Mayonnaise (page 233) plus ½ baked medium sweet potato

PER SERVING:
542 calories,
1,174 IU vitamin D
121 mg calcium
46 g protein
42 g carbohydrates
20 g fat (3 g saturated fat)
1,131 mg sodium
4 g fiber

Halibut with Asparagus and Shiitake Mushrooms and Roasted Potatoes

▶ 1 serving Halibut with Asparagus and Shiitake Mushrooms (page 234) plus ¾ cup roasted diced red potatoes drizzled with 1 teaspoon olive oil and salt and pepper to taste

PER SERVING:
377 calories
607 IU vitamin D
26 mg calcium
41 g protein
38 g carbohydrates
6 g fat (<1 g saturated fat)
512 mg sodium
15 g fiber

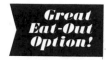

Miso Soup with Tofu and Shrimp and Edamame

PER SERVING:
398 calories
370 IU vitamin D
457 mg calcium
39 g protein
32 g carbohydrates
13 g fat (2 g saturated fat)
972 mg sodium
14 g fiber

▶ 1 serving Miso Soup with Tofu and Shrimp (page 235) plus 1 cup boiled edamame (in the pod)

Eat-Out Tip: A great choice in Japanese restaurants, this will save you money and calories. Combine the miso soup appetizer with the steamed edamame for a light meal.

Broiled Mackerel in Lemon Mint Sauce with String Beans Almondine

PER SERVING:
429 calories
1,011 IU vitamin D
96 mg calcium
30 g protein
12 g carbohydrates
29 g fat (6 g saturated fat)
318 mg sodium
5 g fiber

▶ 1 serving Broiled Mackerel (page 236) plus 1 cup steamed string beans drizzled with olive oil, 1 tablespoon toasted slivered almonds, and salt and pepper to taste

Stuffed Portobello Mushrooms with Roasted Butternut Squash

PER SERVING:
374 calories
804 IU vitamin D
450 mg calcium
20 g protein
36 g carbohydrates
20 g fat (5 g saturated fat)
866 mg sodium
9 g fiber

▶ 1 serving Stuffed Portobello Mushrooms (page 237) plus 1 cup baked butternut squash drizzled with olive oil and sprinkled with cinnamon

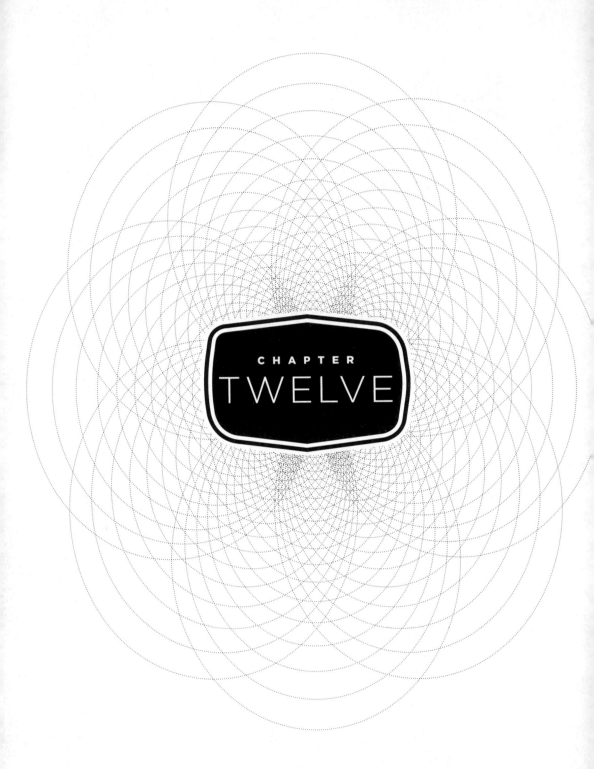

CHAPTER

TWELVE

Summer Light Menus

Summer is the time of year when cravings are low, energy is high, and appetite isn't much of a concern. It's also the time of year when the sun is shining and D levels tend to naturally return to normal for many people. And finally, it's the time of year when you will want lighter fare that you don't have to cook. After all, when it's hot out, who wants to turn on an oven? I sure don't. In the following pages, you'll find options designed specifically for the summer months, so you can keep your D levels high without any unnecessary effort.

Four Features of the Summer Light Plan

1 **ALL OF THESE MEALS ARE RELATIVELY LIGHT ON D.** They are obviously higher in D than you would find elsewhere, but lower when compared them to the winter plan. Depending on your skin color, you probably don't need as much D in the summer as you do in the winter. By providing you with lighter D fare, I've ensured you have more variety in the summer.

2 **THESE MEALS WILL KEEP YOU COOL.** Many require no cooking at all, so you don't have to worry about heating up your kitchen in order to make a meal. Many of these options are also served cold, so they're a refreshing change of pace from the heavier, stick-to-your-ribs winter meals.

3 **THEY PROVIDE LOTS OF VOLUME FOR A MINIMUM OF CALORIES.** These options are all lighter in calories than your winter options. That doesn't mean they are not filling. Many are loaded with low-calorie, high-volume ingredients. You will feel just as satisfied, yet you won't feel weighed down at all.

4 YOU CAN TRANSITION TO SUMMER EATING SEAMLESSLY. As the winter menu does, these menu options work in conjunction with your 4-week plan. You can mix and match them into the meals you are already consuming.

How to Follow the Summer Plan

THE SUMMER PLAN is designed to shake things up, provide a variety of choices, and lighten up your mind-set during the time of year when it's relatively easy to lose weight. Because you are getting plenty of sunlight during the summer, your mood will be better and you'll experience fewer cravings. And the actual temperature of summer works to reduce your appetite because you are too hot to feel like cooking or eating. For best results, follow these pointers.

▶ **IT'S OKAY TO REDUCE YOUR SUPPLEMENT.** You absolutely need a D supplement during the winter months, but the summer is another story. If you have a lighter skin and practice safe sun exposure (roughly 15 to 20 minutes of nonsunscreen sun time a day), you may not need your supplement during the summer.

▶ **WATCH THOSE LIQUID CALORIES.** This can become a problem in warmer months when you're constantly reaching for a cool glass of lemonade or a can of soda. Be aware of how many calories are in that Frappuccino you're grabbing each morning. A soda here and an iced latte there can really put you over your caloric limits quickly and reverse the direction the numbers are headed in on the scale. Keep the 90/10 principle in mind and choose your liquid refreshments carefully. Iced green tea and water are always the best options to help you feel full and hydrate you in the heat.

▶ **IT'S OKAY TO STICK WITH THE FOODS YOU LOVE.** If you love the 4-week plan and it's working for you, you do not have to work in the summer options. They are here for you when you need them, but they are not required.

▶ **MODIFY THE PLAN AS NEEDED.** Summertime often calls for impromptu backyard barbecues and spontaneous trips to the beach. Don't' forget to use the eating out advice and other tips for modifying the plan in Chapter 10.

The Summer Salad Maker

I'M ALL ABOUT great big salads during the summer months. I sometimes eat them twice a day! This is primarily because they are easy. There's no cooking required and very little cleanup. They are also cold and crispy—which is exactly what my taste buds prefer during the hot summer months. And finally, don't let the word "light" fool you. These salads are chock-full of filling ingredients that are incredibly low in calories but high in fiber. They fill you up quickly and keep you satisfied for hours.

Use this formula to customize your own delicious, healthy creations!

THE LIGHT SALAD FORMULA
CHOOSE FROM EACH ROW:

LETTUCE
Fill your plate with one variety or a combo. Lettuce is unlimited.

- Arugula
- Bibb
- Cabbage
- Endive

- Iceberg
- Mesclun
- Mustard greens

- Radicchio
- Romaine
- Spinach

PROTEIN
Top the salad with 4–5 ounces. Bolded items are preferred because they are high in D.

- Beans, ½ cup (chickpeas, kidney, edamame, etc.)
- Chicken or turkey, skinless (baked or grilled)

- **Eggs, hard-cooked** (2)
- **Halibut, baked**
- **Salmon, canned**
- **Shrimp** (about 10 medium)

- **Tofu** (baked or grilled)
- **Tuna, canned**

VEGGIES
Add 1–2 cups of one or more. Sliced mushrooms are preferred.

- Asparagus
- Bell pepper
- Broccoli
- Carrot

- Cauliflower
- Celery
- Cucumber
- **Mushrooms, sliced**

- Onion, red
- Radish
- Tomatoes

TOPPINGS
Add no more than one of the following (optional)

- Apple or pear, sliced (1)
- Artichoke hearts, marinated (3)
- Avocado, ¼–½, sliced

- 2–4 Tbsp Cheese, crumbled, (feta, blue, gorgonzola)
- 1–2 Tbsp Nuts or seeds (sunflower, pumpkin, etc.),

- Olives, halved (5)
- Pasta, ½ cup cooked

DRESSING
Add one:

- 1 tsp olive oil + 2 Tbsp balsamic vinegar
- 2 Tbsp reduced-calorie dressing

- 2 tsp olive oil + lemon juice
- 2 Tbsp lemon juice + Dijon mustard

- 150-calorie serving of any commercially prepared dressing

The Summer Smoothie Maker

AS WITH SALADS, smoothies are also a great summer option. They are easy, portable, and filling—not to mention yummy! The smoothie recipes in this book are all low calorie and most work as snacks, not meals. However, the following smoothie formula is heartier and fit for a meal. Have it for breakfast, lunch, or dinner—whenever it's too hot to cook.

CHOOSE FROM EACH ROW:

PROTEIN *Add one:*	• Cottage cheese, ¾ cup 1% or fat-free • Ricotta cheese, ¾ cup fat-free	• Ricotta cheese, ½ cup reduced-fat • Tofu, 4–5 ounces extra–firm	• Whey protein powder (1 scoop) • Yogurt, 8 ounces fat-free flavored
FRUIT *Add one:*	• Banana (1) • Berries, 2 cups mixed	• Cantaloupe, 2 cups • Honeydew, 1½ cups	• Mango, 1 cup • Watermelon, 2 cups
SWEETENER *Add one:*	• Agave syrup, 1 Tbsp	• Honey, 1 Tbsp • Sugar, 1 Tbsp	
LIQUID *Add one:*	• Kefir, 1 cup nonfat • Milk, 6 ounces, fat-free, D-fortified	• Milk substitute, 6 ounces, D-fortified (soy milk, almond milk, etc.)	• OJ, 6 ounces, D-fortified
FREEBIES *Freebies are unlimited.*	• Cinnamon • Ginger • Ice cubes	• Nutmeg • Tea, unsweet-ened, herbal, green, or black	• Vanilla or almond extract

Summer Menu Plan

Salmon Corn Chowder and Salad

PER SERVING:
457 calories
276 IU vitamin D
254 mg calcium
28 g protein
49 g carbohydrates
17 g fat (4 g saturated fat)
709 mg sodium
8 g fiber

▸ 1 serving Salmon and Corn Chowder (page 239) plus 2 cups mixed greens, 8 cherry tomatoes (halved), ½ sliced cucumber, 2 tablespoons garbanzo beans, 1 tablespoon crumbled feta cheese (optional) tossed with 1 teaspoon olive oil and 2 tablespoons balsamic or red wine vinegar (or 2 tablespoons reduced-calorie dressing), and salt and pepper to taste.

Chilled Salmon Pasta Salad

PER SERVING:
470 calories
529 IU vitamin D
394 mg calcium
35 g protein
36 g carbohydrates
21 g fat (4 g saturated fat)
927 mg sodium
4 g fiber

▸ 4 ounces canned wild salmon (drained and mashed), ⅓ cup asparagus pieces, ¾ cup cooked farfalle pasta, 1 teaspoon capers, 2 teaspoons chopped dill, lemon zest, and salt and pepper to taste, tossed with 1 tablespoon olive oil and lemon juice.

Tuna Salad Niçoise

PER SERVING:
447 calories
285 IU vitamin D
130 mg calcium
40 g protein
25 g carbohydrates
21 g fat (4 g saturated fat)
947 mg sodium
7 g fiber

▸ 4 ounces light tuna packed in water (drained and mashed), over 2 cups mixed greens with 4 olives (pitted and halved), 2 ounces steamed string beans, 2 cooked new potatoes (halved), 1 sliced D-fortified hard-cooked egg, and ½ cup cherry tomatoes drizzled with 1 tablespoon olive oil, 2 tablespoons lemon juice and Dijon mustard whisked together, and salt and pepper to taste.

Oysters on the Half Shell with Gazpacho and Crackers

Great Eat-Out Option!

▶ 6 raw oysters with 1 tablespoon prepared cocktail sauce, horseradish to taste (optional), lemon, plus 1 bowl Gazpacho (page 238) with 120 calories' worth of whole grain crackers (i.e., 1 serving Kashi Heart to Heart Original crackers).

PER SERVING:
349 calories
282 IU vitamin D
150 mg calcium
16 g protein
51 g carbohydrates
13 g fat (1 g saturated fat)
696 mg sodium
12 g fiber

Seared Shrimp with Stir-Fried Vegetables, Brown Rice, and Orange Slices

▶ 1 serving Seared Shrimp with Stir-Fried Vegetables (page 240) plus ¾ cup cooked brown rice and 1 orange, sliced.

PER SERVING:
448 calories
268 IU vitamin D
150 mg calcium
17 g protein
69 g carbohydrates
12 g fat (1 g saturated fat)
878 mg sodium
11 g fiber

Rigatoni with Summer Squash and Mushrooms and Tomato Mozzarella Salad

▶ 1 serving Rigatoni with Summer Squash and Mushrooms (page 241) plus ½ sliced tomato with 1 ounce reduced-fat mozzarella cheese (cubed), drizzled with 1 tablespoon balsamic vinegar and seasoned with salt, pepper, and dried oregano to taste.

PER SERVING:
21 calories
204 IU vitamin D
332 mg calcium
19 g protein
55 g carbohydrates
14 g fat (5 g saturated fat)
570 mg sodium
5 g fiber

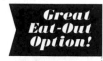

Halibut Tacos with Black Bean Soup

PER SERVING:
445 calories
215 IU vitamin D
147 mg calcium
30 g protein
58 g carbohydrates
12 g fat (2 g saturated fat)
893 mg sodium
12 g fiber

▶ 1 serving Fast and Easy Halibut Fish Tacos (page 242) plus 1 cup low-sodium store-bought black bean soup (i.e., Health Valley Black Bean and Vegetable) or 1 cup any low-sodium soup.

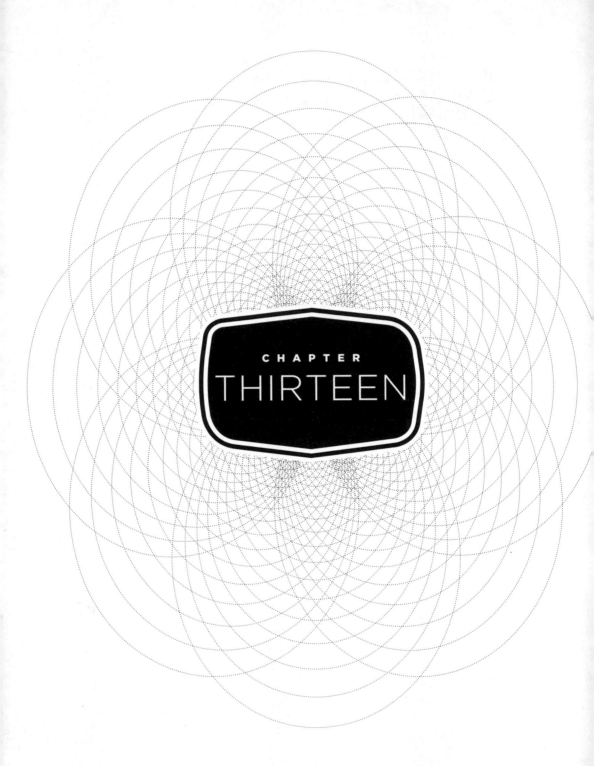

CHAPTER

THIRTEEN

The Slim Down Recipes

In the following pages, you'll find 40 easy-to-make yet mouthwatering recipes, all loaded with at least two power slimmers: D and calcium. Many of them contain several other fat melters, too, ranging from omega-3 fatty acids to protein and more.

Perhaps most important: These recipes don't taste "diet." For that I have Jennifer Iserloh to thank. Better known as "the skinny chef," Jennifer created recipes specifically to be light on calories, but heavy on taste! You won't be disappointed. Some of my new favorites are her Orangetini (perfect when I host my happy hour book club!) and her many smoothie recipes. These recipes have already become staples of mine—and I bet they will for you, too.

MAKE WISE SWAPS. I encourage you to modify the following recipes as needed to suit your taste buds. You don't have to follow any given recipe precisely. It's okay to substitute your favorite spice blend, to use lime juice in place of lemon, and so on. It's also okay to omit various ingredients that you dislike, whether it's peas, collards, or something else. Whenever possible, you don't, however, want to swap out high-D ingredients for low-D ingredients.

MIX IN SEASONAL RECIPES WHEN APPROPRIATE. Most of the recipes listed after the heading 4-Week Slim Down Recipes will work for you at any time of year. Gravitate towards recipes listed under the Winter Warming Menus in the winter and the Summer Light Menus in the summer.

BEWARE OF FLAVOR SIZING. Most of these recipes have been slimmed down. Whole milk has been replaced with fat-free, regular cheese with low-fat, and so on. By slimming down these recipes, I was able to pump up the serving size to keep you fuller, longer. Beware of adding extra oil, butter, or something else. These ingredients can add some serious calories to a recipe and slow your results.

TEACH YOURSELF A FEW AT A TIME. There's no need to make seven new recipes every single week. In my mind, that's a recipe for stress. It's a much better idea to skim through the various recipes, find a few you think you want to try, and then make those over and over again until you get used to them. Then work more variety in from there.

USE THE RIGHT BRANDS. Make sure you are using D-fortified products. Consult the Appendix for a list of recommended brands of margarine, bread, orange juice, and more.

Slim Down Recipes

THE FOLLOWING RECIPES are featured in the 4-Week Slim Down plan. Some of them are also featured in the 7-Day Slim Down. Use them to jump-start your weight loss and continue to lean on these recipes to keep the weight off as you transition to the maintenance plan. Note that some of the beverage recipes work as snacks and others are intended to be meals.

BEVERAGE RECIPES

Bottomless Ginger Mint Iced Tea

Unlimited!

4	green tea bags
¼	cup packed fresh mint leaves, chopped
1	tablespoon freshly grated ginger
	zest and juice of 1 lime

PER SERVING:
7 calories
0 IU vitamin D
10 mg calcium
0 g protein
2 g carbohydrates
0 g fat (0 g saturated fat)
1 mg sodium
0.5 g fiber

Bring 8 cups of water to a boil. Add the tea bags and steep for 4 minutes. Remove the tea bags and discard. Set the tea aside to cool to room temperature, about 30 minutes. Add the mint, ginger, and lime zest and juice. Transfer to an airtight container or pitcher and refrigerate at least 1 hour before serving. Drink throughout the day as needed.

Serves 4   (1 serving = 8 fluid ounces)

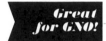

Orangetini

8	**ounces vitamin D-fortified orange juice**
8	**ounces tap water**
4	**ounces vodka**
2	**ounces triple sec**
1	**tablespoon grenadine**
1	**tablespoon orange zest**

PER SERVING:
152 calories
25 IU vitamin D
92 mg calcium
<1 g protein
13 g carbohydrates
0 g fat (0 g saturated fat)
4 mg sodium
0.2 g fiber

In a large pitcher, combine the orange juice, water, vodka, triple sec, grenadine, and orange zest. Stir well. Cover and refrigerate for at least 1 hour before serving.

Serves 4

Hazelnut Latte

2	**cups D-fortified fat-free milk**
2	**teaspoons instant coffee**
2	**teaspoons granulated white sugar**
½	**teaspoon hazelnut extract**

PER SERVING:
134 calories
100 IU vitamin D
403 mg calcium
11 g protein
22 g carbohydrates
0 g fat (0 g saturated fat)
171 mg sodium
0 g fiber

In a small saucepan, combine the milk, coffee, sugar, and extract. Warm over medium heat for 1 to 2 minutes, until the milk steams. Serve immediately.

Serves 2

Chocolate Mocha Smoothie

6	**ice cubes**
6	**ounces D-fortified fat-free milk**
4	**ounces Nasoya TofuPlus extra firm tofu**
4	**teaspoons granulated sugar**
1	**tablespoon unsweetened cocoa powder**
2	**teaspoons instant coffee granules**

PER SERVING:
131 calories
91 IU vitamin D
285 mg calcium
9 g protein
18 g carbohydrates
3 g fat (<1 g saturated fat)
64 mg sodium
2 g fiber

In a blender, combine the ice cubes, fat-free milk, tofu, sugar, cocoa powder, and coffee granules. Blend until smooth and serve immediately.

Serves 2

Fruit Smoothie

1¼	cups D-fortified fat-free milk
¼	cup D-fortified orange juice
¾	cup D-fortified fat-free vanilla yogurt
⅓	cup fat-free whipped topping
½	cup frozen blackberries, strawberries, or raspberries
½	cup frozen cauliflower

In a blender, combine the milk, juice, yogurt, whipped topping, berries, and cauliflower for 1 minute, or until smooth.

Serves 2

Green Tea and Blueberry Smoothie

3	tablespoons water
1	green tea bag
2	teaspoons honey
1½	cups frozen blueberries
½	medium banana
¾	cup calcium-fortified light vanilla soy milk

In a small glass measuring cup or bowl, microwave the water on high until steaming hot. Add the tea bag and allow to steep for 3 minutes. Remove the tea bag. Stir the honey into the tea until it dissolves.

In a blender with ice-crushing ability, combine the berries, banana, and soy milk.

Add the tea to the blender. Blend the ingredients on the highest setting until smooth. (Some blenders may require additional water to process the mixture.) Pour the smoothie into tall glasses and serve.

Serves 2

Kefir Banana Froth

PER SERVING:
225 calories
75 IU vitamin D
241 mg calcium
6 g protein
33 g carbohydrates
0.1 g fat (<1 g saturated fat)
61 mg sodium
0.8 g fiber

1   banana, cut into chunks
2   cups plain nonfat kefir
     Zest of 1 orange
1   cup fresh, D-fortified orange juice
3   tablespoons honey
1   tablespoon lime juice
2   teaspoons vanilla extract
6   ice cubes

In a blender, combine the kefir, orange zest, orange juice, honey, lime juice, vanilla, and ice cubes and puree until thick and smooth. Pair with a piece of fruit, a cheese stick, a hard-cooked egg, or toast with 1 tablespoon of peanut butter for a full meal. Drink only half a serving for a snack.

Serves 4

Creamy Banana Breakfast Smoothie

PER SERVING:
313 calories
182 IU vitamin D
573 mg calcium
19 g protein
51 g carbohydrates
4 g fat (<1 g saturated fat)
129 mg sodium
4 g fiber

6   ounces D-fortified fat-free milk
4   ice cubes
4   ounces Nasoya TofuPlus extra firm tofu
1   medium banana
2   teaspoons granulated sugar
1   teaspoon almond extract

Place the milk, ice cubes, tofu, banana, sugar, and almond extract in a blender. Blend until smooth and serve immediately.

Serves 1

Note: Best used for breakfast, if used for a snack—cut the recipe in half to control calories.

Pineapple Mango Smoothie

- ¾ cup pineapple, cubed
- ½ cup frozen mango
- ¾ cup D-fortified light vanilla soy milk
- 3 tablespoons low-fat cottage cheese
- ¼ teaspoon unsweetened coconut flakes (optional)
- 1 tablespoon ground flaxseed (optional)

PER SERVING:
238 calories
86 IU vitamin D
322 mg calcium
12 g protein
38 g carbohydrates
6 g fat (1 g saturated fat)
239 mg sodium
5 g fiber

In a blender, combine the pineapple, mango, soy milk, and cottage cheese. Blend until smooth. Garnish with the coconut, if using.

Add flaxseed for an extra 2 grams of fiber.

Pair with a piece of fruit, a cheese stick, a hard-cooked egg, or toast with 1 tablespoon of peanut butter for a full meal. Drink only half a serving for a snack.

Serves 1

Almond Smoothie

PER SERVING:
252 calories
75 IU vitamin D
269 mg calcium
6 g protein
41 g carbohydrates
9 g fat (<1 g saturated fat)
136 mg sodium
6 g fiber

- 1 small frozen banana, sliced
- ¾ cup kale, lightly packed, stems removed
- ¾ cup almond milk
- ¾ tablespoon almond butter
- ⅛ teaspoon cinnamon
- ⅛ teaspoon nutmeg
- ⅛ teaspoon ground ginger

In a blender, combine the banana, kale, almond milk, almond butter, cinnamon, nutmeg, and ground ginger. Blend until smooth.

Pair with a piece of fruit, a cheese stick, a hard-cooked egg, or toast with 1 tablespoon of peanut butter for a full meal. Drink only half a serving for a snack.

Serves 1

BREAKFAST RECIPE

PER SERVING:

PER SERVING:
132 calories
277 IU vitamin D
54 mg calcium
12 g protein
5 g carbohydrates
6 g fat (2 g saturated fat)
290 mg sodium
0.8 g fiber

Lox, Eggs, and Onions

1   **teaspoon olive oil**

1   **medium yellow onion, finely chopped**

4   **ounces smoked salmon,* sliced into thin strips**

4   **large D-fortified eggs**

2   **tablespoons D-fortified fat-free milk**

4   **tablespoons sliced scallions**

4   **tablespoons sliced roasted red bell peppers**

Coat a large skillet with cooking spray and place it over medium heat. Add the olive oil. Add the onion and cook for 1 minute. Add the smoked salmon and cook for about 2 minutes, or until the salmon begins to turn opaque and lighter in color. In a small bowl, whisk together the eggs and milk and add them to the skillet. Cook until the eggs are firm and almost dry, about 5 minutes, stirring to heat evenly.

Top each serving with 1 tablespoon each of the scallions and peppers.

Serves 4

*Salmon = Chinook, smoked

LUNCH AND DINNER RECIPES

Turkey Mushroom Burgers

8   ounces fresh D-fortified mushrooms, cleaned

½   onion

3   teaspoons olive oil

1   clove garlic, finely chopped

1   pound fat-free ground turkey

1   tablespoon Worcestershire sauce

1   teaspoon Dijon mustard

   Salt and pepper to taste

PER SERVING:
188 calories
283 IU vitamin D
18 mg calcium
29 g protein
6 g carbohydrates
6 g fat (1 g saturated fat)
208 mg sodium
0.9 g fiber

Finely chop 8 mushrooms, and slice the remaining mushrooms. Finely chop half of the onion half, and slice the other half. Set the sliced vegetables aside.

Heat 1 teaspoon of oil in a nonstick skillet over medium heat. Add the chopped onion and cook for about 6 minutes, or until it's soft. Add the garlic and continue cooking for another minute.

Add 1 teaspoon of the remaining oil. Add the chopped mushrooms and cook for about 5 minutes. Allow the veggies to cool for 5 minutes.

In a large mixing bowl, combine the onion and mushroom mixture, ground turkey, Worcestershire sauce, and mustard. Add salt and pepper to taste. Form into 4 patties. Chill in the refrigerator for about 20 minutes to set.

In the same skillet, heat the remaining 1 teaspoon of oil. Add the sliced mushrooms and sliced onions, and cook until tender, about 5 minutes. Move the mushroom mixture from the pan to a plate. Cover with foil to keep warm.

In the same pan, cook the patties until the internal temperature measures 165°F on an instant-read thermometer or the juices run clear and the meat is no longer pink. Serve them topped with the mushroom and onion mixture.

Serves 4

PER SERVING:
442 calories
280 IU vitamin D
380 mg calcium
23 g protein
65 g carbohydrates
10 g fat (1 g saturated fat)
892 mg sodium
8 g fiber

Spicy Meatballs in Marinara Sauce

1   pack (14 ounces) of Nasoya TofuPlus extra firm tofu

5   ounces fresh D-fortified mushrooms

½   small red or yellow onion

2   cloves garlic, peeled and roughly chopped

1   cup seasoned Italian breadcrumbs

1   D-fortified egg, beaten

¼   teaspoon ground black pepper

2   tablespoons olive oil

1   28-ounce can chopped tomatoes

    Sprig of fresh basil

1   teaspoon crushed red-pepper flakes

8   ounces whole wheat pasta, cooked according to package instructions

Drain and pat the tofu dry. Place it in a large colander and set a heavy small saucepan on top to press it down. Let the tofu drain for about 2 hours. (This can be done the night before. Just store the drained tofu in an airtight container and refrigerate until ready to use.)

Place the mushrooms, onion, and garlic in a food processor and pulse until finely chopped. Transfer to a large bowl. Place the tofu in the food processor and pulse until smooth. Add the tofu, mushroom mixture, breadcrumbs, egg, and pepper to the bowl.

Mix well with your fingers and form 2″ meatballs. Place uncooked meatballs on a sheet of aluminum foil or wax paper. Place a large skillet over high heat and add the olive oil. When the oil is hot, add the meatballs and cook for 2 to 3 minutes, turning occasionally.

Add the tomatoes along with their juices, basil, and red-pepper flakes. Reduce to a simmer. Cook 10 to 15 minutes, covered, until the sauce thickens and the meatballs are cooked through. Serve immediately with the pasta.

Serves 4 (makes 20 meatballs)

Chicken Cacciatore

PER SERVING:
327 calories
272 IU vitamin D
64 mg calcium
32 g protein
33 g carbohydrates
8 g fat (1 g saturated fat)
458 mg sodium
5 g fiber

2	teaspoons olive oil
4	ounces whole wheat pasta
1	pound boneless, skinless chicken breasts, cut into $\frac{1}{2}$" pieces
8	ounces fresh D-fortified mushrooms, quartered
$\frac{1}{2}$	medium red bell pepper, cut into strips
1	small onion, chopped
2	cloves garlic, minced
$\frac{1}{4}$	teaspoon salt
$\frac{1}{4}$	teaspoon ground black pepper
1	can (14$\frac{1}{2}$ ounces) no-salt-added basil-garlic-oregano diced tomatoes
20	large pitted black olives
1	tablespoon finely chopped fresh parsley

In a large nonstick frying pan with a cover, heat the oil over medium-high heat while making the pasta. Add the chicken and cook, turning occasionally, until it's browned on all sides, about 4 minutes. Transfer to a bowl.

Combine the mushrooms, bell pepper, onion, garlic, salt, and pepper in the pan. Reduce the heat to medium, cover, and cook, stirring occasionally, until the mushrooms exude liquid, about 3 minutes. Uncover and cook until most of the liquid evaporates, about 8 minutes.

Stir in the tomatoes with their juice and reserved the chicken with any accumulated juices in the bowl. Reduce the heat to a simmer.

Add the drained pasta to the pan. Add the olives and toss gently to combine. Serve sprinkled with parsley.

Serves 4

PER SERVING:
278 calories
186 IU vitamin D
191 mg calcium
43 g protein
8 g carbohydrates
7 g fat (3 g saturated fat)
564 mg sodium
2 g fiber

Chicken in a Skillet

4	skinless, boneless chicken breast halves, cut into 1″ pieces (about 6 ounces each)
	Salt and pepper to taste
2	cloves garlic, minced
1	can (15 ounces) diced tomatoes, drained
1	bag (5 ounces) baby spinach
2	cups fresh D-fortified mushrooms, thinly sliced
½	cup grated Parmesan cheese

Season the chicken with salt and pepper to taste.

Coat a large nonstick skillet with cooking spray, and place it over medium heat. When it's hot, add the chicken and cook for 5 to 10 minutes, or until it's no longer pink in the middle and the juices run clear.

Remove the chicken to a plate and cover it to keep it warm. Add the garlic to the pan. Cook for 2 to 3 minutes, or until the garlic is fragrant. Add the tomatoes, spinach, and mushrooms. Cook for about 3 minutes, or until the liquid is reduced by half. Put the chicken back in the pan and stir to combine. Adjust the seasoning, if necessary. Sprinkle with the cheese just before serving.

Serves 4

Salmon Burgers

2   cans (about 6 ounces each) wild salmon, drained

2   egg whites, beaten

1   cup whole wheat breadcrumbs

½   cup D-fortified low-fat plain yogurt

½   red onion, minced

1   jalepeño chile pepper, seeded and finely chopped

½   teaspoon ground cumin

1   large tomato, cut into 4 slices

In a medium bowl, mash the salmon with a fork. Add the egg whites, breadcrumbs, yogurt, onion, pepper, and cumin. Stir to blend. Shape into 4 burgers.

Coat a nonstick skillet with cooking spray. Place the skillet over medium heat and cook the burgers for 6 minutes, turning once, or until browned and crisp.

Place each salmon burger over bed of field greens and top with a tomato slice.

Serves 4

PER SERVING:
259 calories
409 IU vitamin D
345 mg calcium
27 g protein
24 g carbohydrates
6 g fat (1 g saturated fat)
585 mg sodium
2 g fiber

Tuna Tacos

1	teaspoon ground cumin
1	teaspoon chili powder
½	teaspoon garlic powder
½	teaspoon salt
¼	teaspoon ground black pepper
4	tuna steaks (4 ounces each)
1	avocado
¼	cup loosely packed fresh cilantro leaves
¼	cup light sour cream
1	tablespoon lime juice
8	corn tortillas
½	white onion, thinly sliced

Combine the cumin, chili powder, garlic powder, ¼ teaspoon of the salt, and pepper in a bowl. Rub this mixture over the tuna steaks and let them stand for 10 minutes.

Meanwhile, in a food processor, combine the avocado, cilantro, sour cream, lime juice, and the remaining ¼ teaspoon of salt. Puree until smooth.

Preheat a ridged grill pan that has been coated with cooking spray. Add the tuna and cook for 2 to 3 minutes per side, or until well-marked and cooked through. Transfer to a cutting board. Thinly slice the tuna.

In a skillet, heat the tortillas over a gas burner, turning occasionally, for about 1 minute, or place the tortillas between clean paper towels and microwave them on high for 15 to 20 seconds to warm. Fill the tortillas with sliced tuna and onion and top them with the cilantro-avocado cream.

Serves 4

Puttanesca Pizza

PER SERVING:
332 calories
242 IU vitamin D
235 mg calcium
30 g protein
39 g carbohydrates
7 g fat (2 g saturated fat)
652 mg sodium
7 g fiber

1	pound uncooked whole wheat pizza dough, defrosted (i.e., Trader Joe's 100% Whole Wheat Pizza Dough)
1	can (28 ounces) no-salt-added diced tomatoes
3	cans (5 ounces each) light tuna in spring water, well drained
5	ounces thinly sliced fresh D-fortified mushrooms
½	red onion, thinly sliced
⅓	cup chopped, pitted, good-quality black olives
¼	cup fresh basil leaves, chopped
½	teaspoon crushed red-pepper flakes
1½	cup grated part-skim mozzarella

Preheat the oven to 425°F. Coat a 19" x 12" baking sheet with cooking spray. Roll out the pizza to fit the cookie sheet and let it rise for 15 minutes.

Drain the tomatoes and spread them over the pizza crust. Sprinkle the tuna, red onion, olives, basil, and red pepper over the tomatoes. Sprinkle the cheese evenly over the top and bake 10 to 15 minutes, until the cheese is bubbly and begins to brown. Cool for 5 minutes before slicing into 6 equal servings.

Serves 6

PER SERVING:
185 calories
156 IU vitamin D
87 mg calcium
16 g protein
30 g carbohydrates
1 g fat (<1 g saturated fat)
752 mg sodium
11 g fiber

Miso Glazed Shrimp and Shiitake Mushrooms

2	ounces Eden Foods dried shiitake mushrooms
2	tablespoons white or red miso paste
1	tablespoon reduced-sodium soy sauce
1	tablespoon rice wine vinegar
2	teaspoons granulated white sugar
1	teaspoon ground black pepper
10	ounces fresh shiitake mushrooms, stems removed and discarded
1	head broccoli
½	pound medium shrimp, tails removed
4	scallions, thinly sliced

Place the dried shiitakes in a small bowl with ½ cup boiling water. Soak for 15 to 20 minutes. Remove the mushrooms and set them aside. Place a coffee filter over a coffee cup and strain the soaking liquid to remove any sediment. Place the liquid in a small saucepan. Chop up the rehydrated mushrooms and set them aside.

Place the miso paste, soy sauce, vinegar, sugar, and pepper in the saucepan with the mushroom liquid. Whisk until smooth. Place over low heat along with the chopped and sliced rehydrated mushrooms. Cook over low heat for about 5 minutes, until the mushrooms are soft and some of the liquid has reduced.

Heat a large grill pan over high heat. Set out the fresh mushrooms, broccoli, and shrimp and coat them with a thick layer of cooking spray. Turn them over and coat the other side with another layer of cooking spray, and place them on the grill. Grill for 4 to 6 minutes, turning once or twice, until the mushrooms are soft, broccoli is tender, and the shrimp are cooked through. Transfer to a large bowl and add the miso mixture. Toss to coat. Garnish with the scallions and serve immediately.

Serves 4

Penne with Mushrooms and Artichokes

PER SERVING:
323 calories
267 IU Vitamin D
104 mg Calcium
12 g protein
50 g carbohydrates
10 g fat (2 g saturated fat)
193 mg sodium
11 g fiber

6	ounces whole wheat penne
1	tablespoon olive oil
8	ounces fresh D-fortified mushrooms, sliced
1	onion, chopped
3	cloves garlic
16	cherry tomatoes, halved
1	cup artichoke hearts, drained and chopped
¼	cup reduced-fat pesto
4	teaspoons grated Romano cheese

Bring a large pot of lightly salted water to a boil. Add the penne and cook according the package directions. Drain.

Meanwhile, heat the oil in a large nonstick skillet over medium-high heat. Add the mushrooms and onion and cook, stirring occasionally, for 7 to 8 minutes, or until the mushrooms have released their liquid and start to brown slightly. Add the garlic and cook for 1 minute longer. Stir in the tomatoes and artichoke hearts and cook for another 1 to 3 minutes, or until the tomatoes just begin to soften.

Add the pasta and toss to combine. Remove from the heat and stir in the pesto.

Divide among 4 bowls and top each serving with 1 teaspoon of the cheese.

Serves 4

PER SERVING:
303 calories
187 IU vitamin D
523 mg calcium
20 g protein
23 g carbohydrates
14 g fat (1 g saturated fat)
174 mg sodium
8 g fiber

Szechuan Eggplant and Tofu

2	packs (14 ounces each) of Nasoya TofuPlus extra firm tofu
1/2	cup cold water
1	tablespoon reduced-sodium soy sauce
2	teaspoons sugar
1	teaspoon ground black pepper
1	tablespoon Chinese black vinegar* or balsamic vinegar
2	teaspoons finely minced ginger
2	cloves garlic, minced
1	teaspoon crushed Szechuan peppercorns* or crushed red-pepper flakes
1	teaspoon cornstarch
2	tablespoons sesame oil
1	pound small purple or Asian eggplant,* cut into 1/2" cubes
1/2	head broccoli, cut into florets
1	small white onion, peeled and cubed
4	scallions, thinly sliced

*Available at Asian grocery stores.

Drain and pat the tofu dry. Place it in a large colander and set a small, heavy saucepan on top of it. Drain for about 2 hours; it will become more compact as it drains.

In a small bowl, combine the water, soy sauce, sugar, pepper, vinegar, ginger, garlic, peppercorns or red-pepper flakes, and cornstarch. Set it aside. Heat a large skillet over high heat. Add the sesame oil, eggplant, broccoli, and the onion to the skillet. Cook for 3 to 4 minutes, stirring often until the vegetables start to brown. Reduce the heat to low. Whisk the soy sauce mixture until smooth, then add it to the skillet. Add the tofu and gently stir. Cook for about 1 minute until a light sauce forms. Turn the heat off and garnish with the scallions. Serve immediately.

Serves 4

Portobello Mushroom Barley

2	teaspoons olive oil, preferably extra virgin
1	cup fresh sliced D-fortified portobello mushrooms, chopped
¼	cup sliced scallions
1	bay leaf
½	teaspoon minced fresh or crumbled dried rosemary
¼	teaspoon salt
⅛	teaspoon ground black pepper
½	cup instant barley
¾	cup low-sodium chicken broth
2	teaspoons balsamic vinegar

Coat a wide, shallow saucepan or skillet with cooking spray. Set over medium-high heat for 1 minute. Add the oil and swirl to coat the pan. Heat for 1 minute. Add the mushrooms, scallions (reserve a few greens for garnish, if desired), bay leaf, rosemary, salt, and pepper. Stir. Cover and cook, stirring frequently, for 2 minutes, or until the mushrooms give off liquid.

Add the barley. Cook, stirring, for 2 minutes, or until the barley is coated with the seasonings. Add the broth and bring to a boil.

Cover and cook over medium-low heat for about 10 minutes, or until the barley is tender. Remove and let stand, covered, for a few minutes, or until all of the liquid is absorbed and the flavor develops.

Remove and discard the bay leaf. Stir in the vinegar. Serve, garnished with the reserved scallion greens (if using).

Serves 4

PER SERVING:
120 calories
142 IU vitamin D
17 mg calcium
5 g protein
20 g carbohydrates
3 g fat (<1 g saturated fat)
168 mg sodium
5 g fiber

PER SERVING:
252 calories
333 IU vitamin D
29 mg calcium
6 g protein
33 g carbohydrates
11 g fat (1 g saturated fat)
169 mg sodium
3 g fiber

Brown Rice Mushroom Pilaf

1	cup reduced-sodium, fat-free chicken broth
½	cup water
½	cup pecans
1½	tablespoons olive oil
1	large onion, halved and thinly sliced
2	cloves garlic, minced
10	ounces fresh D-fortified mushrooms, quartered
½	teaspoon dried thyme
¼	teaspoon salt
¾	cup short- or long-grain brown rice

Preheat the oven to 350°F. Combine the broth and water in a small saucepan and bring to a boil over high heat. Set aside.

Toast the pecans in a large nonstick skillet over medium heat, stirring often, for 3 to 4 minutes, or until lightly browned and fragrant. Tip onto a plate.

In a large ovenproof saucepan or casserole with a lid, heat the oil over medium heat. Add the onion and garlic. Cover and cook, stirring often, for about 6 minutes, or until tender.

Stir in the mushrooms, thyme, and salt (the pan will seem dry). Cover and cook, stirring often, for about 6 minutes, or until the mushrooms have released their liquid and the liquid has evaporated. Stir in the rice and pecans.

Add the reserved broth mixture and bring it to a boil. Cover the saucepan or casserole and transfer it to the oven. Bake for 50 to 60 minutes, or until the rice is tender and the liquid has been absorbed. Let stand for 5 minutes before fluffing with a fork and serving.

Serves 4

WINTER WARMING RECIPES

THE FOLLOWING RECIPES are loaded with D, and packed with total-body warmth. These meals seriously satisfy during the time of year when you want something thick, hearty and substantive.

Beef Barley Soup

1	tablespoon olive oil
1	pound well-trimmed lean, boneless beef top round, cut into ¾" cubes
2	medium onions, halved and thinly sliced
3	cloves garlic, minced
¾	teaspoon salt
¼	teaspoon ground black pepper
½	teaspoon dried thyme, crumbled
10	ounces fresh D-fortified portobello mushrooms, sliced
2	ribs celery with some leaves, thinly sliced
2	medium carrots, sliced
1	medium parsnip, halved lengthwise and sliced
3	cups water
3½	cups fat-free beef broth
½	cup pearl barley
	Chopped fresh parsley or dill (optional)

PER SERVING:
369 calories
338 IU vitamin D
77 mg calcium
32 g protein
36 g carbohydrates
12 g fat (4 g saturated fat)
700 mg sodium
8 g fiber

Heat the oil in a Dutch oven or a large, heavy saucepan over medium heat. Add the beef cubes. Lightly brown the beef until the liquid evaporates. Add the onions and garlic and cook for 3 to 5 minutes, or until the onions soften. Add the salt, pepper, and thyme and cook for 1 minute. Add the mushrooms and cook for 3 minutes, or until the mushrooms begin to soften. Add the celery, carrots, and parsnip and stir for 2 minutes. Add the water and the broth and simmer for 45 minutes. Stir in the barley and simmer for 45 minutes longer, or until the barley is soft. Sprinkle with fresh parsley or dill, if using.

Serves 4

Wild Mushroom and Beef Stew

PER SERVING:
372 calories
638 IU vitamin D
205 mg calcium
39 g protein
32 g carbohydrates
11 g fat (4 g saturated fat)
537 mg sodium
6 g fiber

- ¼ teaspoon salt
- 1 pound lean cubed stew beef, trimmed of excess fat
- ¼ cup whole wheat flour
- 2 tablespoons paprika
- ⅛ teaspoon ground cayenne
- ½ teaspoon ground black pepper
- 2 tablespoons Smart Balance Light Buttery Spread
  Nonstick cooking spray
- 1 large onion, peeled, sliced into thin rings
- 4 cloves garlic, minced
- ½ cup tomato paste
- 4 cups reduced sodium, fat-free beef broth
- 1 pound fresh D-fortified mushrooms, quartered
- 1 pound kale, thinly sliced
- 2 tablespoons fresh parsley, chopped

Sprinkle the meat with salt. On a sheet of wax paper, mix the flour, paprika, cayenne, and black pepper. Roll the beef into the flour mixture. Set aside.

Heat a stockpot over medium-high heat. Add the Buttery Spread and the beef and cook 3 to 5 minutes, turning once or twice until the beef is golden. Remove the beef to a plate.

Add a light layer of cooking spray. Add the onions and garlic and cook 4 to 5 minutes until the onions begin to soften and brown. Add a tablespoon of water if they begin to stick. Add the tomato paste and cook 1 additional minute.

Return all the meat and any accumulated juices to the stockpot. Add the broth, scrapping up any browned bits and spices from the bottom of the pot. Stir in the mushrooms. Cover and simmer 2 to 2½ hours, until meat is fork tender. Add the kale during the last 10 minutes of cooking. Spoon into warm soup plates and garnish with parsley.

Serves 4

Chicken Scallopini with Garlic Mushroom Sauce

4	thin raw chicken cutlets (about 1 pound)
1/2	teaspoon salt
1/4	teaspoon ground black pepper
1/2	cup flour
2	teaspoons paprika
1	tablespoon olive oil
1	tablespoon D-fortified soft tub margarine (i.e., Smart Balance Light Buttery spread)
10	ounces fresh D-fortified mushrooms, sliced
4	cloves garlic, minced
1/2	cup white wine
1/2	cup fat-free reduced-sodium chicken broth
	Juice of 1 lemon
1/4	cup flat parsley leaves, chopped

Sprinkle both sides of the chicken with the salt and pepper. Place the flour and paprika on a sheet of wax paper and mix with your fingertips. Dredge the chicken in the flour mixture and transfer the cutlets to a fresh piece of wax paper.

Heat a large skillet over medium-high heat. Add the oil and chicken cutlets. Cook for 3 to 4 minutes per side, turning once. Transfer the chicken to a clean plate. Add the margarine, mushrooms, and garlic. Cook for 1 to 2 minutes, stirring often, until the mushrooms begin to soften. Add the wine and cook for 1 minute, until the liquid reduces. Add the chicken broth and return the chicken to the skillet. Cook for an additional minute, turning the chicken once to coat it in the sauce. Add the lemon and parsley and serve immediately.

Serves 4

PER SERVING:
260 calories
389 IU vitamin D
22 mg calcium
28 g protein
13 g carbohydrates
8 g fat (2 g saturated fat)
518 mg sodium
2 g fiber

PER SERVING:
409 calories
628 IU vitamin D
110 mg calcium
37 g protein
14 g carbohydrates
23 g fat (5 g saturated fat)
341 mg sodium
5 g fiber

Sesame-Crusted Salmon

1	teaspoon toasted sesame oil
4	Pacific wild salmon fillets (5 ounces each)
1/2	cup black sesame seeds
1/4	cup reduced-fat sour cream
1	teaspoon wasabi powder
1	tablespoon freshly squeezed lime juice
12	ounces green beans, trimmed
1	tablespoon reduced-sodium soy sauce

Preheat the oven to 400°F. Brush a small baking dish very lightly with some of the sesame oil.

Pat the fillets dry with a paper towel. Spread half of the sesame seeds on a small plate and press both sides of the fish firmly onto the seeds. Transfer the fillets to the prepared dish. Bake for 10 minutes, or until the fish flakes easily with a fork.

Combine the sour cream, wasabi, and lime juice in a small bowl. Thin with a few drops of water, if necessary, to make a smooth sauce. Set aside.

Heat the remaining oil in a large nonstick skillet over medium-high heat. Working in batches, if necessary, add the green beans, stirring often, and cook until the beans are lightly browned. Stir in the soy sauce and the remaining 1/4 cup of sesame seeds.

Divide the green beans among four plates. Top each with a piece of salmon and drizzle the reserved wasabi sauce around the plate.

Serves 4

Orange Poached Salmon with Star Anise and Spinach

PER SERVING:
331 calories
800 IU vitamin D
244 mg calcium
39 g protein
20 g carbohydrates
10 g fat (1 g saturated fat)
214 mg sodium
2 g fiber

2	cups D-fortified orange juice
1	1" piece ginger, peeled and thinly sliced
2	star anise pods*
1	tablespoon black peppercorns
4	wild salmon fillets, skin on (about 1½ pounds)
2	cups packed baby spinach leaves, thinly sliced
1	cup orange sections
½	red onion, minced

Place the orange juice, ginger, star anise, and peppercorns in a medium saucepan. Bring to a boil. Add the salmon filets and cover. Turn off the heat and let the salmon cook in the liquid for 10 minutes, or until it is cooked through and flakes when pressed with a fork. Remove the salmon and peel off the skin. Set aside.

Remove and discard the ginger, star anise, and peppercorns from the orange juice mixture. Bring the orange juice to a simmer over medium-low heat and cook for 4 to 6 minutes, until it reduces by half. Turn the heat off. Add the spinach and cover to wilt it. Once the spinach is wilted, divide it among four plates and top with the sauce. Top each spinach mound with one piece of the salmon. Divide the orange sections and the minced onions among the four plates as a garnish and serve immediately.

Serves 4

*Use the whole pod, available at local grocery stores.

PER SERVING:
486 calories,
1,174 IU vitamin D
101 mg calcium
46 g protein
29 g carbohydrates
20 g fat (3 g saturated fat)
1,095 mg sodium
2 g fiber

Catfish Fingers with Spicy Mayonnaise

½	cup reduced-fat mayonnaise
1	tablespoon tomato paste
1	tablespoon hot sauce
1	cup seasoned whole wheat or white breadcrumbs
¼	cup yellow cornmeal
2	pounds wild catfish fillets, cut into strips about 4" long
¼	teaspoon salt
2	D-fortified eggs
1	tablespoon olive oil

In a small bowl, mini-chopper, or blender, mix the mayo with the tomato paste and hot sauce. Blend until smooth. Set aside.

On a piece of wax paper or aluminum foil, mix the breadcrumbs and cornmeal with your fingertips. Sprinkle the fish with the salt. In a shallow dish, beat the eggs. Dip the fish strips into the egg and then coat them in the breadcrumb mixture. Transfer to a plate.

Coat a large skillet with cooking spray and place it over high heat. Add the olive oil. Brown the fish strips on one side, cooking for 3 to 4 minutes, or until the breadcrumb coating is crispy and golden. Turn the fish sticks and cook an additional 3 to 4 minutes, or until the fish is no longer translucent and is cooked through. Serve immediately with the spicy mayonnaise.

Serves 4

Halibut with Asparagus and Shiitake Mushrooms

PER SERVING:
279 calories
607 IU vitamin D
26 mg calcium
39 g protein
23 g carbohydrates
2 g fat (<1 g saturated fat)
490 mg sodium
15 g fiber

¼	pound Eden Foods dried shiitake mushrooms
4	halibut fillets (6 ounces each)
12	asparagus spears, woody ends removed
1	tablespoon grated fresh ginger
2	tablespoons mirin (sweetened rice wine) or sake
2	tablespoons low-sodium soy sauce
	Salt and pepper

Place the mushrooms in a small bowl with ½ cup of boiling water. Soak for 15 to 20 minutes. Remove the mushrooms and set them aside. Place a coffee filter over a coffee cup and strain the soaking liquid to remove any sediment.

Preheat the oven to 400°F. Set four 12″ squares of aluminum foil on a counter and place a fillet in the middle of each one. Evenly divide the mushrooms, asparagus, and ginger on top of the fish.

In a small bowl, combine the soy sauce and mirin and season with a small pinch of salt and black pepper. Drizzle the mixture over the fillets.

Fold the foil over the ingredients and crimp the edges to seal. Place the packets on a large baking sheet and bake for 20 to 25 minutes, depending on the thickness of the fillets.

Serves 4

Miso Soup with Tofu and Shrimp

2	ounces Eden Foods dried shiitake mushrooms
15	ounces low-sodium chicken or vegetable broth
2	cups water
1	package (14 ounces) Nasoya TofuPlus extra firm tofu, drained
½	pound small shrimp, such as rock shrimp, peeled and deveined
5	ounces baby spinach
4	ounces D-fortified fresh Monterey mushrooms, thinly sliced
3	tablespoons low-sodium miso paste
4	scallions, thinly sliced

Rinse the dried mushrooms well under cold running water. In a large saucepan over high heat, heat the broth and water. As soon as it comes to a boil, turn the heat off, add the mushrooms, and cover. Set aside and soak the mushrooms for 15 minutes.

Cut tofu into small cubes and add them to the soup. Simmer the tofu for a few minutes on low heat. Add the shrimp, spinach, and fresh mushrooms, and cook for 1 minute more, until the spinach has wilted, the mushrooms are soft, and the shrimp is cooked through.

Transfer ½ cup of the broth to a small bowl. Whisk in the miso paste. Gradually return the miso mixture to the soup. Stir the soup gently. Turn off the heat and add the scallions. Serve immediately.

Serves 4

Broiled Mackerel

2	tablespoons D-fortified soft tub spread (Smart Balance Light Buttery Spread)
1	tablespoon chopped fresh mint
1½	teaspoons lemon juice
½	teaspoon ground black pepper
4	skinless mackerel fillets (5 ounces each)
¼	teaspoon salt

Place the broiler rack 2" to 3" from the heat source and preheat the broiler.

In a small bowl, combine the spread, mint, lemon juice, and ¼ teaspoon of the pepper.

Season the fish with the salt and the remaining ¼ teaspoon of pepper. Lightly coat a broiling pan with cooking spray and arrange the fish on it. Broil, without turning, until the top is lightly browned and the flesh is completely opaque, 5 to 6 minutes. Spread the lemon-mint butter evenly over the fish and serve.

Serves 4

PER SERVING:
316 calories
1,011 IU vitamin D
20 mg calcium
26 g protein
0.5 g carbohydrates
22 g fat (5 g saturated fat)
314 mg sodium
0 g fiber

Stuffed Portobello Mushrooms

2	tablespoons canola oil
1	pound Swiss chard, trimmed, stems removed and sliced crosswise, and leaves chopped
2	cloves garlic, crushed
½	teaspoon salt
1	bunch scallions (about 6), bulbs and greens separated and sliced
8	D-fortified fresh portobello mushroom caps
½	cup drained canned fire-roasted diced tomatoes
5	ounces part-skim mozzarella or smoked mozzarella, coarsely grated
2	tablespoons finely chopped fresh parsley
	Ground black pepper
¼	cup crushed, unsalted, roasted cashews

Heat the oven to 400°F. Heat 1½ teaspoons of the oil in a large skillet over medium-high heat. Add the chard stems, garlic, and salt, and cook for 5 minutes. Stir in the scallion bulbs and chard leaves. Cook until tender, about 12 minutes, stirring occasionally. Remove from heat.

Coat the mushrooms with the remaining 4½ teaspoons of oil and lightly sprinkle all over with salt. Put the mushrooms on large baking sheet.

Stir the tomatoes, scallion greens, cheese, and parsley into the cooked chard mixture and season with black pepper to taste. Fill the mushrooms with chard stuffing. Bake until hot, 15 to 20 minutes. Sprinkle with the cashews before serving.

Serves 4

SUMMER LIGHT RECIPES

USE THE FOLLOWING recipes during the summer months, when your appetite is light and you don't need to eat as much D as you do in the winter.

Gazpacho

2	cups grape tomatoes, halved
2	tablespoons chopped celery
2	tablespoons chopped red bell pepper
2	tablespoons chopped onion
2	tablespoons chopped cucumber with skin
1	tablespoon chopped cilantro
2	tablespoons ground flaxseed
	Wedge of lime
	Pinch of salt
1	cup ice water
	Hot-pepper sauce

In a blender or food processor, combine the tomatoes, celery, bell pepper, onion, cucumber, cilantro, flaxseed, squeeze of lime juice, salt, and ¼ cup of the water. Pulse for 1 to 2 minutes, or until the mixture is finely chopped. Add up to ¼ cup more water and pulse to combine. Season to taste with the hot-pepper sauce.

Serves 1

PER SERVING:

348 calories
93 IU vitamin D
396 mg calcium
17 g protein
36 g carbohydrates
14 g fat (2 g saturated fat)
619 mg sodium
9 g fiber

Salmon and Corn Chowder

1	tablespoon olive oil
1	small white onion, chopped
5	slices low-sodium turkey bacon, chopped
2	stalks celery, chopped
1	tablespoon flour
1	teaspoon Old Bay seasoning
¼	teaspoon salt
¼	teaspoon ground black pepper
¼	teaspoon ground red pepper
15	ounces fat-free, low-sodium chicken or vegetable broth
1	large baking potato (about ½ pound), peeled and cubed
2	cups fresh corn kernels or frozen corn kernels
1	cup D-fortified fat-free milk
2	salmon fillets, skin removed (about 8 ounces), cut into 1″ chunks
2	tablespoons half-and-half
½	cup chopped chives

Place a large stockpot over medium-high heat. Add the oil. Add the onion, bacon, and celery. Cook for 5 to 6 minutes, until the onion begins to soften but not brown. Add the flour, Old Bay, salt, black pepper, and red pepper. Cook an additional 2 to 3 minutes, stirring continuously until the flour coats the onion and starts to stick to the bottom of the pan without browning. Decrease heat to low.

Add the broth and potato cubes. Bring to a boil. Cover and simmer 15 to 20 minutes until the potato cubes are tender. Mash the potato cubes directly in the pot. Add the corn and milk. Simmer 1 to 2 minutes, stirring often, until the corn is tender and the mixture thickens. Turn the heat off and add the salmon. Cover and let rest for 3 minutes to allow the fish to cook through. Stir in the half-and-half and sprinkle with chives and serve.

Serves 4

Seared Shrimp with Stir-Fried Vegetables

PER SERVING:
234 calories
534 IU vitamin D
83 mg calcium
14 g protein
21 g carbohydrates
11 g fat (1 g saturated fat)
879 mg sodium
5 g fiber

2	ounces peeled and deveined medium shrimp
	Salt and pepper
1	teaspoon canola oil
1	tablespoon lime juice
2	teaspoons crushed fresh ginger
1	teaspoon cornstarch
1	teaspoon minced garlic
1	teaspoon toasted sesame oil
1	cup broccoli florets
½	cup snow peas
½	cup grated carrots
½	cup fresh D-fortified mushrooms, sliced
2	teaspoons low-sodium soy sauce
2	tablespoons water

Season the shrimp to taste with salt and pepper. Heat the canola oil in a large, heavy skillet over high heat. The pan should be as hot as possible. Place the shrimp in the pan and sear for 45 to 60 seconds. Remove and set aside.

In a large bowl, blend the lime juice, ginger, cornstarch, garlic, and sesame oil until the cornstarch is dissolved. Mix in the broccoli, peas, carrots, and mushrooms, tossing to lightly coat. In the same pan used for the shrimp, cook the vegetables for 2 minutes, stirring constantly. Stir in the soy sauce and water. Cook for about 10 minutes, or until the vegetables are crisp-tender.

Place the vegetables on a plate and top with the shrimp.

Serves 1

PER SERVING:
323 calories
201 IU vitamin D
98 mg calcium
12 g protein
49 g carbohydrates
9 g fat (2 g saturated fat)
242 mg sodium
4 g fiber

Rigatoni with Summer Squash and Mushrooms

8	ounces rigatoni pasta
2	tablespoons olive oil
1	medium yellow or green summer squash, halved lengthwise and sliced (about 2 cups)
2	cups fresh D-fortified mushrooms, sliced
½	cup sliced carrots (1 small)
½	cup sliced scallions, all parts (about 6 scallions)
2	tablespoons chopped fresh dill
½	teaspoon crushed red-pepper flakes
¼	teaspoon salt
¼	cup grated Parmesan cheese

Cook the pasta according to the package directions. Scoop out ½ cup of pasta-cooking water and reserve. Drain the pasta and return it to the cooking pot to keep warm.

Meanwhile, in a large nonstick skillet over medium-high heat, warm the oil. Add the squash, mushrooms, and carrot. Toss to mix. Cover and cook, stirring occasionally, for 3 to 4 minutes, or until tender-crisp. Add the scallions. Cook for about 2 minutes, or until the carrots are tender and the scallions are wilted. Add the dill, pepper flakes, and salt. Remove from the heat.

Add the pasta to the vegetable mixture. Moisten with a few tablespoons of the reserved cooking water. Add the cheese. Toss over low heat for about 1 minute, or until the cheese melts. Serve warm or at room temperature.

Serves 4

Fast and Easy Halibut Fish Tacos

PER SERVING:
335 calories
215 IU vitamin D
87 mg calcium
26 g protein
34 g carbohydrates
12 g fat (2 g saturated fat)
414 mg sodium
7 g fiber

1	small white onion, thinly sliced
½	Jalapeño chile pepper, finely chopped, wear plastic gloves when handling
1	tablespoon lime juice
1	tablespoon chopped fresh cilantro
½	teaspoon salt
1	tablespoon canola oil
1	pound halibut fillet
1	teaspoon chili powder
1	teaspoon ground cumin
8	corn tortillas
2	cups shredded romaine lettuce
1	medium tomato, chopped
1	avocado, sliced

In a medium bowl, combine the onion, chile pepper, lime juice, cilantro, and ¼ teaspoon of the salt.

Heat the oil in a large nonstick skillet over medium-high heat. Sprinkle the halibut with the chili powder, cumin, and the remaining ¼ teaspoon salt. Add to the skillet and cook until the fish flakes easily with a fork, 5 to 6 minutes per side. Remove from the skillet.

Heat the tortillas according to the package directions. Fill the tortillas with the halibut, lettuce, tomato, and avocado. Top with the onion mixture.

Serves 4 (2 tacos each)

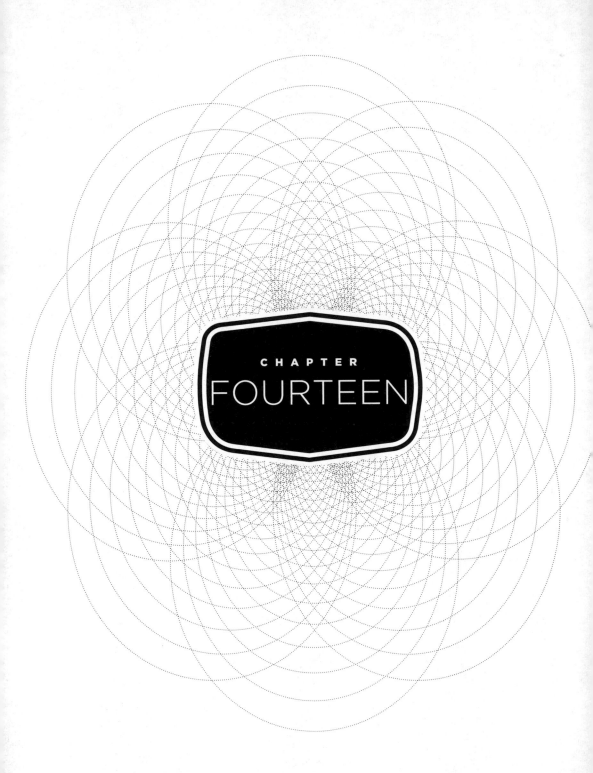

CHAPTER

FOURTEEN

Speed Slimming Moves

Many people think that there is only one right way to exercise. They assume that you must follow a complex set of instructions precisely or you won't see results. But this just isn't true. Yes, there are a few things that will help to make your fitness routine more effective, and you will learn what those are within the pages of this chapter. But one magic secret? That's nonsense. There are many ways to slim down.

I used to sign up for fitness classes—spinning, kick boxing, you name it. I wanted to sculpt my body into a sexy little shape. With every class, I'd start off with lots of motivation. But soon, my attendance waned. My excuses grew more and more lame—and finally, I would just be too embarrassed to show up after missing so many sessions.

Eventually, however, I realized that the real problem was that I disliked being indoors. I never have to talk myself into exercising outdoors. In fact, sometimes I don't even think of it as exercise! I love the sensation of the wind in my hair or cool air on my face when I go running. I love being alone with my thoughts. I even love the people I see along the way—the old guy who always waves, or the woman who comments about how my dog is taking me for a run rather than the other way around.

Why should I force myself to exercise indoors so I can try the latest, hottest exercise class when I can much more easily motivate myself to go for a run? There's no reason. None.

It's the same for you. The best exercise is the exercise you will do. Period. In the end, the most important ingredient in your fitness routine is your willingness to participate. If you hate your routine, you're either going to skip your workouts or you're going to do them halfheartedly. That's just not effective.

In the following pages, you'll find many routines and exercise suggestions. Some are intense. Others, not so much. Some you can do at home. Others you'll have to do at the gym. I tried to include several options so you could find at least one that works for your lifestyle. If you're really a newbie, I'll also teach you the psychological know-how you need to get yourself to start an exercise plan and stick with it. But first, I want to explore several myths that might be standing between you and fitness success.

MYTH #1:

YOU DON'T HAVE TO EXERCISE TO SHED FAT. ALL YOU HAVE TO DO IS EAT LESS.

THERE ARE SOME diet plans that don't require any exercise. They say that you don't need it. And to some extent, this is true. You can lose weight just by dieting. The problem with this is that dieting tends to cause your body to lose a combination of fat and muscle protein. Depending on the composition of your diet, you might lose a lot of muscle and only a little fat. A higher-protein food plan that is rich in vitamin D and a few other key nutrients (like this plan!) will help you preserve muscle mass so your body burns more fat and less muscle.

That said, the best way to preserve muscle mass is to use it. Your muscles were designed to move, and when you move them more than usual they grow denser, firmer, and stronger. This is a good thing because muscle is calorie-hungry tissue. Every pound of it burns 35 to 50 calories a day, even at rest. Muscle tissue is an incredibly important part of your metabolism. Without it, everything slows down and the only way to keep losing weight is to keep eating less food.

Here are eight more compelling reasons to get moving.

YOU'LL FEEL LIKE FOLLOWING THE DIET. Many dieters cheat or quit because of stress eating. Regular exercise boosts production of the brain's endorphins, feel-good chemicals that numb pain and boost mood. It also reduces stress, increases self-confidence, and reduces symptoms of depression and anxiety.

YOU'LL GAIN CONTROL OVER EMOTIONAL EATING. Exercise lifts mood, keeps you busy, and can even provide a social outlet that makes you less lonely, too. All of this makes you a lot less likely to resort to a tub of popcorn, two chocolate bars, and movies on demand after a hard day at the office.

YOU'LL PREVENT THE WINTER BLUES. Research suggests that burning off 350 calories—the equivalent of roughly 3.5 miles of walking—three times a week can reduce symptoms of depression about as effectively as antidepressants.

YOU'LL HAVE A LOT MORE ENERGY. Exercise helps to improve sleep, which, in turn, fuels you with the energy you need for the next day. Exercise also improves your muscle strength, boosts your endurance, and keeps your cardiovascular system working more efficiently. When your heart and lungs work more efficiently, you have even more energy to get through your busiest days.

YOU'LL BE MORE LIKELY TO KEEP OFF WHAT YOU LOSE. Research consistently shows that people who exercise 20 to 35 minutes a day are more likely to maintain their weight loss. In one study done on 97 women, fewer than 1 percent of participants who exercised regained tummy fat during the year after a diet, compared to 25 percent of study participants who didn't exercise.

YOU'LL FEEL BETTER ABOUT YOUR BODY. Studies suggest that simply seeing fitness improvements, like running a faster mile or lifting more weight than before, can improve your self-esteem and body image. And this is seriously important. Researchers have shown time and time again that people who lose weight for health reasons are a lot more likely to be successful than people who attempt to lose weight purely because of vanity. And people who feel more confident about their bodies at the beginning of a weight-loss program are much more likely to lose weight and keep it off than people who are ashamed of their bodies. I want you to stand proudly in front of the mirror and love what you see!

IT CAN REPLACE "EATING" AS A SOCIAL ACTIVITY. Various studies have shown that most of us are about as fat as the people we hang out with. That's because eating can be induced by peer pressure. You know what I'm talking about. You are having just one drink with a girlfriend after work. Then she orders a cheese plate along with some nachos and won't let up with the, "Oh come on. You're not going to help me eat all of this? Really? You're no fun anymore!"

Instead of meeting for drinks, try connecting with friends during a group running session, on a hike, or on your way to yoga class.

YOU PRIME YOUR BODY FOR FAT BURNING. When you exercise regularly, levels of fat burning enzymes go up—and these enzymes become more effective, too. This allows your muscles to more easily harvest and burn fat for fuel.

MYTH #2:
YOU ARE ALLERGIC TO EXERCISE.

THIS LINE'S STRAIGHT out of my good friend Andi's mouth. About a year ago, she told me, "I am allergic to exercise. It doesn't matter what you tell me to do. I'm going to hate it."

She said this right before the two of us took a long walk through town as we window-shopped and people-watched. We probably walked about 2 miles, but she didn't think of it as exercise because she was having such a good time. (And I'm a good enough friend that I did not point out that fact!)

Still, I get it. I understand where Andi and many other people are coming from when they say they are allergic to exercise. Starting and maintaining an exercise plan can be frustrating and difficult. Yet, it's my firm belief that hating exercise is a lot like hating certain foods. Think of all the foods you once hated when you were younger. I had a long list, including tomatoes, beans, and spinach. Why did I hate them? Because, as a kid, I thought they looked and smelled funny, so I refused to try them.

Then, periodically, over the course of my life, I tried those foods. I now love all of them. Tomatoes, in particular, are among my favorites—especially when they are in season. I even have a tomato garden in my yard. As a kid I hated them because they were new to me. The thought of not liking them was a lot worse than the actual experience of eating them.

Exercise is the same. Often, the dread of it is worse than the actual experience. If you continually tell yourself things like, "I have to exercise" and "let's get this over with," you will dread it even more. On the other hand, if you tell yourself, "I want to exercise today," what do you think might happen? Try it. You might realize that it's really not that bad after all.

Here's another suggestion: Give it 2 weeks. The first couple weeks of any exercise program are the hardest. That's because your body just isn't used to making those movements. Everything feels foreign and awkward. You might even feel embarrassed, as if other people might be looking at you and thinking that you are doing it wrong. And this is also the time period when many people feel delayed onset muscle soreness.

After a couple weeks, however, things will change. Your muscles develop what's known as muscle memory. That means that you no longer have to use your brain to tell your muscles to do the grapevine during a dance class. Your legs just do the movement without you thinking about it.

This muscle memory will take longer to develop for some types of exercise than others, based on how complicated the exercise is and how often you practice, but it always develops. Once it does, exercise doesn't feel so foreign and hard.

Finally, exercise can actually be enjoyable if you don't think of it as exercise. My friend Andi had so much fun strolling along she never considered the fact that she walked 2 miles that day. Think of it as movement. Do you enjoy walking your dog? Or riding a bike with your child? Or playing *Just Dance* on the Wii? These are all forms of movement that will get you in shape, and they all count—as exercise!

MYTH #3:

EXERCISE ERASES OVEREATING.

THIS MYTH IS particularly problematic, and it can really stand in the way of your success. It's true that each mile you walk or run burns 50 to 100 calories. Those burned calories speed weight loss and they do serve as a mild caloric buffer for those times when you go a little overboard. But they are no substitute for reasonable eating.

Here's why. The typical craving-induced binge can quickly set you back 1,000 calories or more. For instance, just one slice of pie at a typical restaurant will run you 400 calories. Add some ice cream and you've got 200 more. That's 600 calories right there, and we're only talking about dessert. To work that off, you'd need to run or walk 6 miles. That's a lot, and few people ever do it.

Exercise is important for all of the reasons I've stated. But don't use it as a crutch to deal with overeating. If you do, you'll end up disappointed in your progress.

MYTH #4:

EXERCISE MAKES YOU HUNGRY.

MANY PEOPLE THINK that exercise makes you hungry, causing you to overeat and undo all of the calorie burning you accomplished during your session. Researchers in the United Kingdom recently proved this theory wrong. They studied 12 men and women, tracking their energy expenditure and food intake for 16 days. The researchers asked the participants to complete various types of workouts on different days, ranging from no exercise at all to very high intensity exercise. The participants were hungrier when they exercised, but that hunger did not cause them to undo their calorie burn. They only compensated for about 30 percent of the calorie deficit caused by exercise. In other words, 70 percent of the calories they burned during exercise stayed burned. Other research done in Australia found that 12 weeks of an exercise program (about 25 miles of walking or running a week) made study participants feel hungrier just before meals, but participants remarked that they also felt satisfied more quickly.

YOU MUST SPEND AN HOUR AT THE GYM AND SERIOUSLY EXHAUST YOURSELF TO GET RESULTS.

I USED TO fall prey to this myth. I thought that I needed to hit the gym four or five times a week, do set after set of weights, and sweat like crazy to "feel the burn."

It wasn't until I met New York fitness trainer Pete Cerqua, author of *The 90-Second Fitness Solution*, that I changed my mind. Pete challenged me to do something completely counterintuitive: exercise less. He said there was no reason for me to lift weights more than 1 day a week or do more than one set of any exercise. Yes, heavy weights were good, but I didn't even need to fully fatigue any given muscle—thus inducing major muscle soreness the following day. He just wanted me to lift for about 90 seconds per exercise.

At first I thought he was nuts. Then I tried it and I actually got stronger. Here's why: Finally, I was lifting consistently. In trying to do the multiple sets and multiple weight lifting workouts per week, I was expecting too much of myself. I just couldn't keep up such a regimen. I didn't have the time or the inclination, so I would do it for a while and then I would stop and then I would start and then I would stop. As a result, I never really got into great shape.

Once I switched to Pete's less-is-more weight lifting model, I got in shape and I stayed there.

But you may be wondering about studies or articles you might have read about how more sets and days are better. You know what? All of those studies were done on body builders. If it's your goal to grow the kind of serious muscle that makes you look like a female version of the Incredible Hulk, then sure—more sets and days at the gym are in order. If your goal is to firm up and melt fat, the one-day-a-week, one-set-and-you're-done model is much more appropriate. Sound good?

Create the Perfect Plan for You

In the following pages, you'll find six different exercise programs. Pick and choose from among them to assemble a surefire plan that you don't mind doing and can maintain. You might do just one entire exercise prescription. You might decide to incorporate several. The choice is yours. Just remember: Keep it realistic. The more suited it is to your lifestyle, the more likely you'll keep it up.

EXERCISE PRESCRIPTION #1:

THE MORNING WALK

MANY PEOPLE ATTEMPT to exercise in the afternoon and evening, after they've gotten their to-do lists completed. This is tough because most to-do lists have a way of expanding and oftentimes end up encroaching on exercise time. During the afternoon and evening, most people are quite tired, too. It's really easy to find excuses not to move when you're tired.

Enter the morning: The perfect time of day to move. The morning is the time of day most under your control. It's also a great way for you to get in a little fresh air and mood-boosting sunlight so the rest of your day goes a little easier. The morning walk is especially important during the winter months, when sunlight disappears after about 4 o'clock. Although it won't provide your body with very much D (due to the angle of the sun), it will still give you a needed mood and energy boost. It will also help to improve sleep later on. Research done at the Fred Hutchinson Cancer Research Center in Seattle found that women who took 1-hour morning walks were more likely to sleep better than women who didn't walk.

As a bonus, most people, myself included, find that they feel better all day long when they move in the morning. I have fewer cravings, less stress, and more focus at work. But perhaps most important is this: A morning walk sets the tone for the rest of the day. Once you get in a little activity in the morning, you'll have more willpower to stick to your goals for the rest of the day. Indeed, a morning walk is one of the best things you can do for your overall mood and productivity.

IF YOU OPT FOR THE MORNING WALK PRESCRIPTION:

MAKE THIS A NONNEGOTIABLE PART OF YOUR DAY. Nothing happens until you get that walk in. Once you are done with your walk, you can eat breakfast, check e-mail, or make a phone call. But the day doesn't start until you move.

WALK WITH A PURPOSE. If you can, tie your morning walk to something else you have to do anyway. That way, you'll be more likely to do it every day. For instance, I walk my daughter to school. You can also walk to a coffee shop rather than drive or just walk your dog rather than let your dog out into the yard. Your dog will thank you and probably help to remind you to do it the following day!

WALK OUTDOORS IF YOU CAN. You'll get a bigger mood boost from walking in sunlight than you will from doing it indoors on a treadmill.

GO WITHOUT SUNSCREEN ON YOUR ARMS AND LEGS IF YOUR WALK WILL LAST LESS THAN 15 MINUTES. Always wear sunscreen on your face, though. The vitamin D produced in your skin is powerful and effective—but exposure to both UVA and UVB rays can be deadly for your skin, so you don't want to expose it for any longer than 15 minutes. If you are very light skinned and burn easily, wear sunscreen at all times.

CARDIO THREE TIMES A WEEK

CARDIO IS A great way to burn calories, boost mood, and improve your heart health. Intense cardio can also help you shed stress and might even reduce hunger and cravings.

IF YOU OPT FOR THE CARDIO PRESCRIPTION:

CHOOSE CARDIO YOU ENJOY. Don't force yourself to do exercise routines that you don't love. Only do exercise that you can embrace—forever. So if you once loved tennis, find a nearby court and a partner. If you once loved to swim, get in the pool. If you love being social, Zumba or another group dance class might be your thing. The point is to pick something that you can look forward to. That's true even if you've picked a gym for its hot tub or steam room because it feels so good after your workout.

PAIR EXERCISE WITH SOMETHING ELSE YOU LOVE. Let's say that every time you exercise, you meet a good friend. This friend becomes your walking partner, running partner, or tennis partner. If you only see this friend when you exercise together, you will start to look forward to your exercise sessions because you can't wait to talk to your friend. Similarly, if you love being outside, then be active outside. Or, if you love music, invest in an iPod Nano and upload your favorite tunes, then make sure it's clipped to you every time you head to the gym.

EASE INTO IT. As I've said, many people end up hating exercise because they've tried before to go from zero fitness to 100 percent fitness all in the same day. They get off the couch, put on some sneakers, and try to run up and down stadium steps for an hour. They are not used to getting their heart rate up that high, and their muscles are not used to working that hard. As a result, the entire experience is painful from start to finish. Worse, they feel sore the next day and dead tired afterward.

When done correctly, exercise should not hurt. Unless you are training for the Olympics, you should not feel as if someone has just sucked all of the available oxygen out of your body. It should not leave you feeling sore or immobilized the next day, either. When running hurts, that's when I know something is wrong—and it's usually that my shoes need to be replaced.

So, especially if you haven't exercised in a while, ease into it. Be gentle with yourself. Exercise just 1 day a week at first. Then, when you are feeling fitter, progress to 2 days a week, and then 3. If you slowly ease into it like this, you'll slowly build your fitness and you'll be able to avoid most of the discomfort of getting in shape.

EXERCISE PRESCRIPTION #3

STRENGTH TRAIN AT HOME 1 TO 2 TIMES A WEEK

STRENGTH TRAINING BUILDS muscle, and muscle burns calories. Every pound of muscle in your body burns 35 calories a day just to maintain itself. The more muscle you have, the more calories your body burns—even during sleep. Your metabolism also kicks into high gear during the 24 hours after a workout, as your body repairs your muscles and restocks your fuel stores.

Starting on page 257, you will find two different workout routines that can be done at home. Pick the routine that works best for you.

NO EQUIPMENT

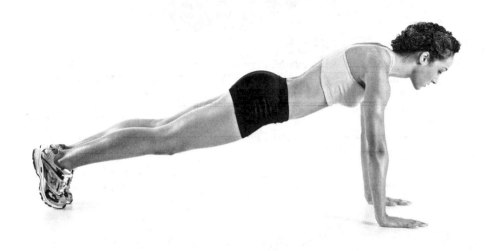

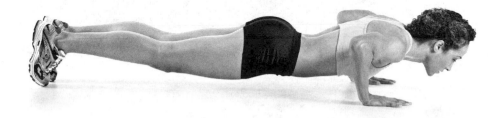

PUSHUP

Start on all fours with your palms on the floor under your shoulders and your legs
extended. (Note: If you are not yet strong enough for a Big Girl–style pushup, rest
your knees on the floor, lift your calves, and cross your ankles.)

Lower your body until your chest nearly touches the floor. Pause and then return
to the starting position. Repeat up to 90 seconds.

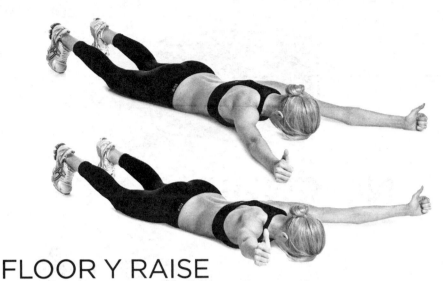

FLOOR Y RAISE

Lie facedown. Extend your arms overhead at a 30-degree angle to your body, with your palms facing in, forming the shape of a Y. (For variety, you can also do this exercise with your arms out to your sides in the shape of a T or directly overhead in the shape of an I. The different arm positions work slightly different areas of your upper back.)

Lift your arms as high as you can. Pause and then return to the starting position. Repeat 90 seconds.

IIIIIIIIIIIIIIIIIIIIIIIIIIIIIIIIIIIIIIIIIIIIIIIIIIIIIIIIIIIIIIIIIIIIIIIIIIIIIIIIIIIIIIIIIIIIIIIIIIIIIIIIIIIIIIIIIIIIIIIIIIIII

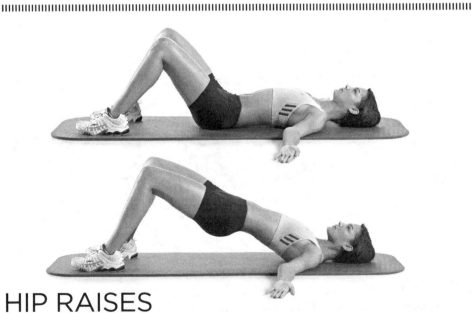

HIP RAISES

Lie on your back with your knees bent and feet flat.

Raise your hips so your body forms a straight line from your shoulders to your knees. Hold for up to 90 seconds. (Note: To increase the intensity of this exercise, extend one leg, holding for 45 seconds on each side.)

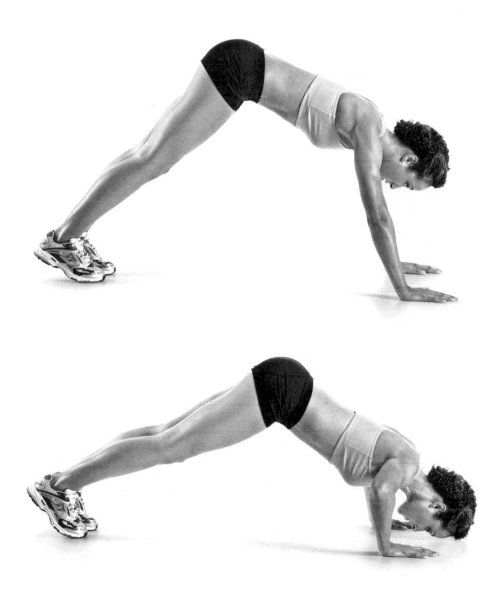

INVERTED PRESS

Bring your body into a downward facing dog position with your hips in the air and your body weight evenly distributed between your hands and feet. Your body should form a triangle and your hands should be shoulder-width apart.

Keep your body in this position as you bend your elbows and bring your head almost all the way to the floor. Pause and then return to the starting position. Repeat up to 90 seconds.

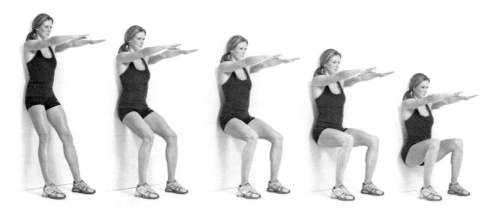

WALL SQUAT

Lean your back against a wall with your feet about shoulder-width apart and slightly forward from the wall.

Keeping your back against the wall, bend your knees and slide down the wall a few inches. Hold for 10 seconds.

Then lower yourself a few more inches. Hold for 10 seconds.

Then lower yourself a few more inches. Hold for 10 seconds.

Then a few more inches. Hold for 10 seconds.

Then do the whole sequence in reverse, repeating once.

||||||||||||||||||||||||||||||||||||||||||||||||||||||||||||||||||||||||||||||||||||||||||||||||||||||||||||||||||||||||||||||||||||||||||||||||||||||||||||

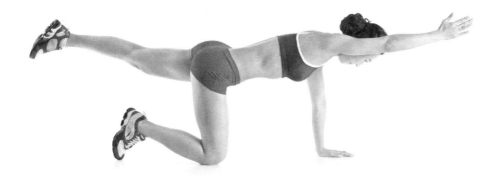

BIRD DOG

Get on all fours. Extend your right arm and left leg. Hold for 5 seconds. Lower and repeat with your left arm and right leg. Keep switching sides for a total of 9 reps on each side.

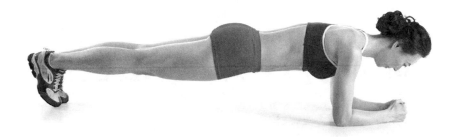

PLANK

Start in a modified pushup position with your elbows bent and your forearms against the floor. Your body should form a straight line from your shoulders to your ankles. Brace your core by tightening your abs. Hold for up to 90 seconds.

IIIIIIIIIIIIIIIIIIIIIIIIIIIIIIIIIIIIIIIIIIIIIIIIIIIIIIIIIIIIIIIIIIIIIIIIIIIIIIIIIIIIIIIIIIIIIIIIIIIIIIIIIIIIIIIIIIIIIIIIIIIIIIIIIIIIIII

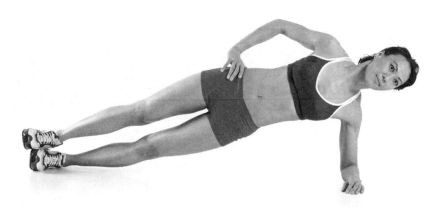

SIDE PLANK

Lie on your left side with your knees straight. Prop your upper body on your left elbow and forearm.

Tighten your abs and raise your hips until your body forms a straight line from your ankles to your shoulders.

Breathe deeply and hold for up to 45 seconds. Repeat on the other side.

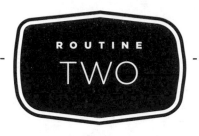

ROUTINE

TWO

WITH DUMBBELLS

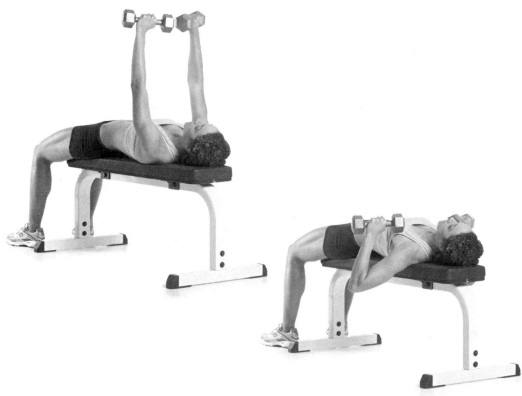

DUMBBELL BENCH PRESS

Lie on your back on a flat bench. If you do not own a weight lifting bench, you can use a piano stool or something similar. Extend your arms and hold the dumbbells over your chest so they are nearly touching.

   Lower the dumbbells to beside your chest. Pause and then push the weights back up to the starting position. Repeat up to 90 seconds.

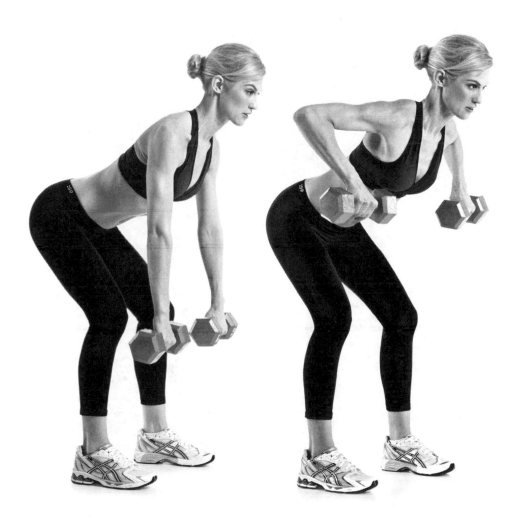

DUMBBELL ROW

Grab a pair of dumbbells. From a standing position, bend at your knees and lean forward from your hips until your torso is almost parallel with the floor. Extend your arms toward the floor.

Bend your arms and pull the dumbbells up to your sides. You should feel your shoulder blades pinching closer together as you do this. Pause and then return to the starting position. Repeat for 90 seconds.

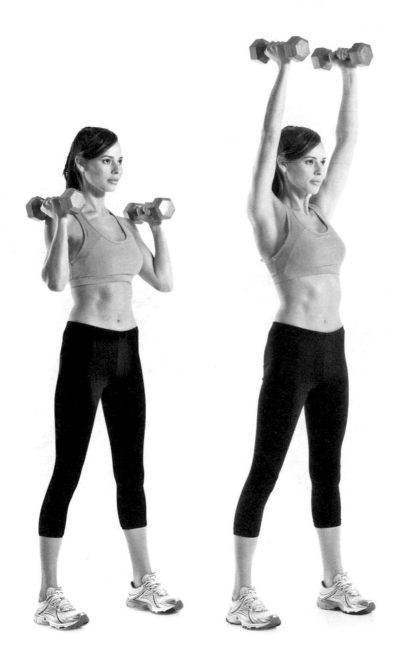

SHOULDER PRESS

Stand with a pair of dumbbells at shoulder level, your elbows bent, and palms facing in. Your feet should be shoulder-width apart and your knees should be slightly bent.
    Press the dumbbells directly overhead until your arms are completely extended. Pause and then return to the starting position. Repeat for up to 90 seconds.

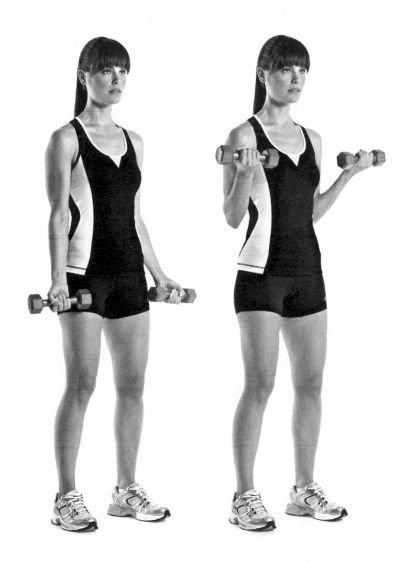

DUMBBELL CURL

Stand with your arms extended by your sides, palms forward.

Bend your elbows and curl the dumbbells up to your shoulders. Keep your upper arms close to your sides the whole time. Pause and then return to the starting position. Repeat for up to 90 seconds.

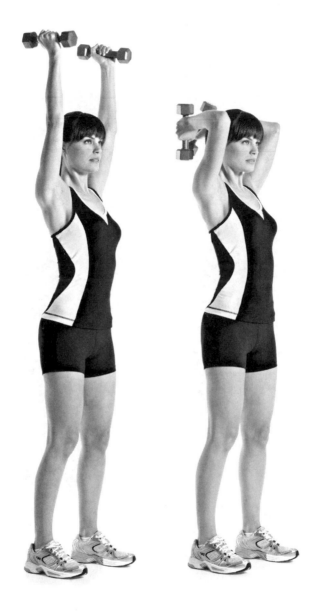

OVERHEAD TRICEPS EXTENSION

Stand with your arms extended overhead and your feet shoulder-width apart. Face your palms toward one another, holding a dumbbell in each hand.

Keeping your upper arms in place, lower the dumbbells behind your head. Pause and then return to the starting position. Repeat for up to 90 seconds.

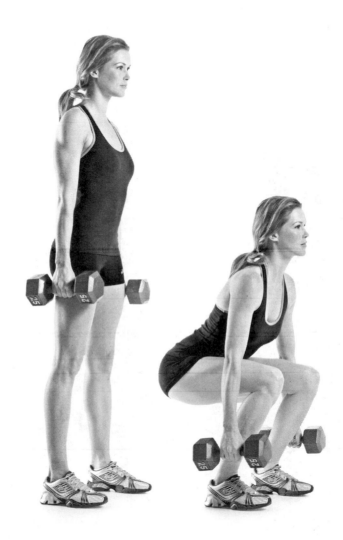

DUMBBELL SQUAT

Stand while holding a pair of dumbbells at your sides. Your palms should be facing in.
Bend your knees and lower into a squat, pushing your hips back and bringing your thighs parallel with the floor. Pause and then return to the starting position. Repeat for up to 90 seconds

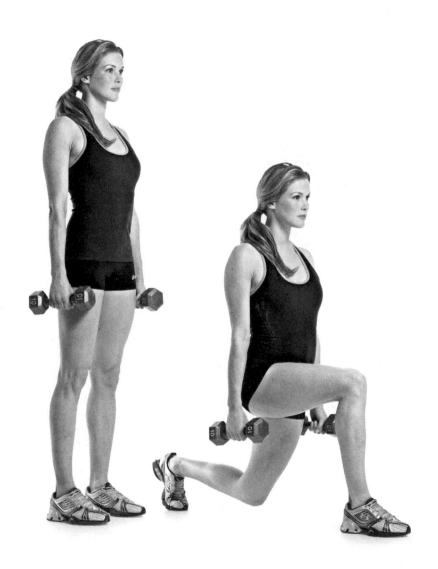

DUMBBELL LUNGE

Stand with your feet shoulder-width apart and dumbbells at your sides.

Step forward with your right leg. Slowly lower your body until your front knee is bent 90 degrees.

Pause and then push back to the starting position. Repeat for up to 90 seconds, alternating legs.

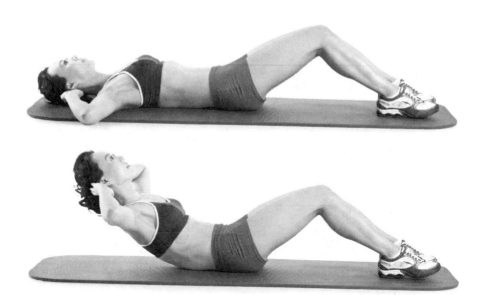

CRUNCH

Lie on your back with your knees bent and your feet on the floor. Place your fingers behind your ears and rest your elbows out to the sides.

Lift your head and shoulders as you crunch your rib cage toward your pelvis. Pause and then return to the starting position. Repeat for up to 90 seconds.

DUMBBELL SIDE BEND

Stand with a pair of dumbbells overhead, your arms extended and in line with your shoulders.

Without twisting your upper body, bend directly to your left as far as you can. Pause and then return to the starting position. Then bend to the right. Repeat for up to 90 seconds.

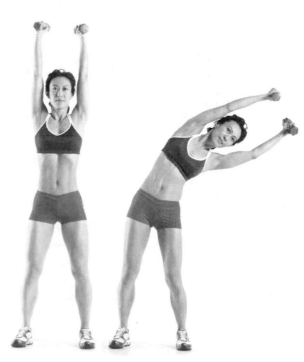

STRENGTH TRAIN AT THE GYM 1 TO 2 TIMES A WEEK

IF YOU'D RATHER train at the gym, here are several options. Choose one of the following:

▶ Perform the dumbbell routine shown on pages 262 to 269. It also works at the gym with dumbbells or barbells.

▶ Take a strength class such as Bodypump or Power Yoga.

▶ Do the circuit, moving from machine to machine. Work through the circuit doing 8 to 12 lifts (as heavy as you can) on the chest press, chest fly, row, low back extension, biceps curl, triceps push, and shoulder press. For your legs, do a wall sit (back against a wall, knees bent at 90 degrees) for 90 seconds. For your abs, do a plank for 90 seconds plus 10 to 20 crunches on a fitness ball

GATHER MOVEMENT AS YOU GO

I CALL THIS the sneaky lifestyle movement because you reap the benefits of exercise while doing the kinds of things you must do anyway, such as straightening your house and doing yard work. But don't feel as if you are cheating if you opt for this prescription. Sneaky exercise can really add up. Depending on how much of it you work into a given day, you can burn up to 750 additional calories every day! Use these pointers.

DO: WEAR A PEDOMETER. Clip it to your waistband to count your steps for you. On average, sedentary people take only 2,000 to 3,000 steps a day. Adding 2,000 steps will help you maintain your current weight and stop gaining weight. If you add more than that, your extra steps can help you drop pounds.

DO: ERRANDS ON FOOT. Or on a bike. Try to keep your car parked—or parked far away—as often as possible. You'll be amazed how many things you can get done on foot or on a bicycle if you are creative about it. I use the basket on the front of my bike to carry everything from bank deposit slips to mail to items I purchase at the convenience store.

DO: MORE BY HAND. Sweep grass or leaves off the street with a broom, rather than with a leaf blower. Use a nonmotorized vacuum for small cleaning jobs. Hang clothes on a line rather than using the drier. All of these things not only help you burn calories, they also will cut your electric bill and help you do your part to reduce your carbon footprint.

EXERCISE PRESCRIPTION #6

GATHER MOVEMENT YOGA OR STRETCHING BEFORE BED

FEW PEOPLE TRULY relax before bed, which results in poor sleep (or lack of sleep). As I've mentioned a few times before, poor sleeping habits can make it difficult to lose weight. The less sleep you get, the hungrier and grumpier you feel, which makes it tough to stick to a healthy eating plan.

If you tend to toss and turn at night or wake repeatedly, I highly recommend you stretch, do gentle yoga, or practice some other form of relaxation before bed, such as meditation or deep breathing.

If you opt for yoga, you'll get an extra mindfulness boost that might carry over into your eating habits. One study, done at Deakin University in Australia, found that a 12-week yoga program that included postures, breathing, relaxation, and meditation helped women reduce binge eating and improve self-esteem and body image. They all lost weight, too.

If you opt for yoga, you can take a class in the evening or do a series of poses on your own at home. Just make sure to do a gentle form of yoga. Something like Power Yoga is more of a strength and cardio workout and will rev you up rather than help you to unwind.

In the following pages, you'll find some gentle stretches to try in the evening before bed.

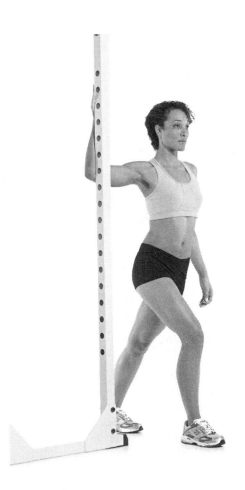

DOORWAY
STRETCH

Bend your arm at a 90-degree angle in a high-five position. Place your forearm against a door frame. Step through the doorway with your right foot until you feel a comfortable stretch in your chest. Hold for 15 to 20 seconds and then switch sides.

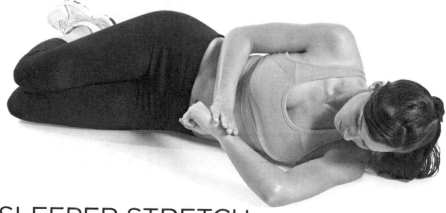

SLEEPER STRETCH

Lie on your left side with your left upper arm on the floor and your elbow bent at 90 degrees. Adjust your torso so that your right shoulder is slightly behind your left and your left forearm is pointing toward the ceiling. Gently push your left hand toward the floor until you feel a comfortable stretch in the back of your left shoulder. Hold for 15 to 20 seconds and then switch sides.

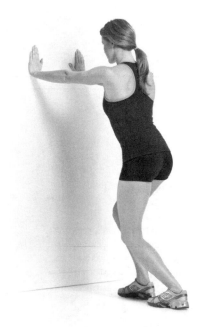

WALL PUSH

Stand about 2 feet in front of a wall with one leg in front of the other. Place your palms against the wall and lean forward. Press down through your back heel until you feel a stretch in your calf. Hold for 2 seconds, release, and repeat 10 times. Repeat on the other side.

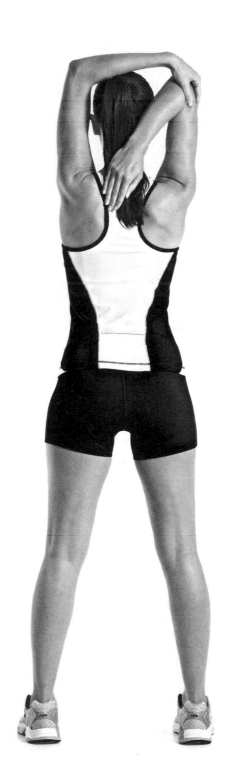

TRICEPS
STRETCH

Stand or sit. Reach overhead
with your right arm, bending
your elbow as if you were
attempting to scratch your left
shoulder blade.

Grasp your right elbow with
your left hand. Pull your right
arm behind your head and to
the left until you feel a stretch.
Hold for 15 to 20 seconds and
then repeat on the other side.

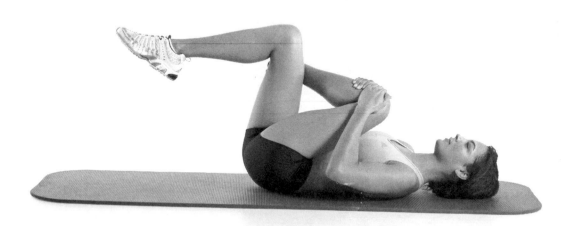

STANDING HAMSTRING STRETCH

Place your right foot on a bench or chair. Extend your leg until it is completely straight. With your left leg slightly bent, lean forward until you feel a stretch. Hold for 15 to 20 seconds and then switch legs.

||||||||||||||||||||||||||||||||||||||||||||||||||||||||||||||||||||||||||||||||||||||||||||||||||||||||||||||||||||||||||||||||

GLUTE STRETCH

Lie on your back with your knees bent and feet flat on the floor. Cross your left leg over your right so that your left ankle sits over your right thigh. Grab your left knee with both hands and pull it toward the middle of your chest until you feel a stretch. Hold for 15 to 20 seconds and then repeat on the other side.

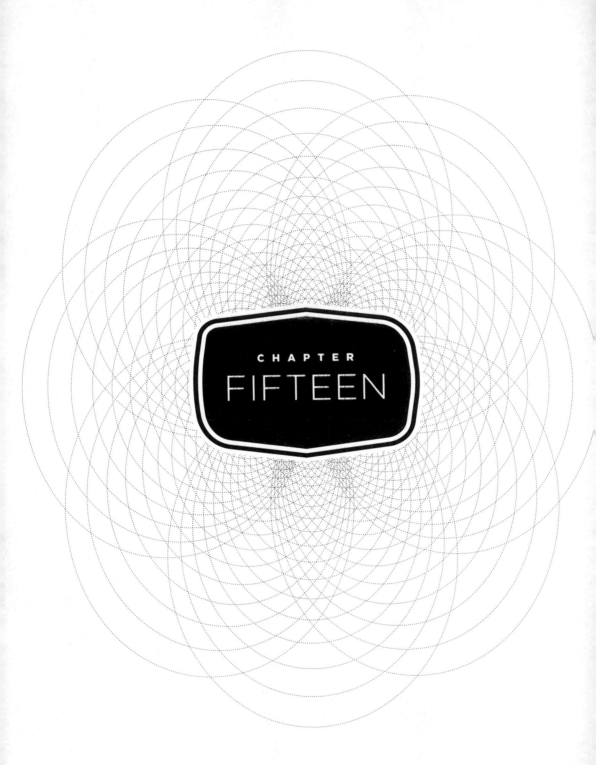

CHAPTER

FIFTEEN

How to Stay Slim for Life

A s I've said previously, I really want this to be the last diet you ever start. I want you to finally reveal the slim, toned, gorgeous shape that's there inside you!

As a result, I offer a different approach than what you may have tried in the past. If you reached your goal weight on a low-carb plan, there was a scary moment when you had to add the carbs back in without going overboard. If you followed a calorie-counting diet, then you had to increase your calories to maintain, rather than lose—but not too much! It was a stressful and frustrating experience, especially if you had lost weight but then saw the numbers on the scale start to rise.

Fortunately, with this plan you didn't cut anything out, so there's nothing to add back in. You didn't give up meat. You didn't give up carbs. You didn't give up fat. You didn't even give up sugar or alcohol or coffee. So, this time, you don't have to worry about having that fearful moment when you "break" the diet and have your first taste of something that you've been craving for months because you've been eating in a balanced way all along.

Indeed, all you need to do to keep the weight off for life is this: Transition from following the 7-Day Slim Down to living it. That's what this chapter is all about, helping you to shift from thinking of this plan as a temporary fix and to thinking about it as the nutrition plan you will be following for life.

And there are at least four compelling reasons to turn the 7-Day Slim Down into a rest-of-your-slim-and-sexy-life.

Four Reasons to Become a Lifer

UNLIKE OTHER DIETS you might have tried, there's absolutely no reason to go off this diet and plenty of reasons to stay on it—for life. Following are four of them.

YOU'LL LIVE LONGER. Unlike some other popular diets, you don't have to worry about the 7-Day Slim Down raising your cholesterol, saddling you with heart disease, or giving you a case of constipation that just won't quit. To the contrary, this diet is loaded with foods that fuel both weight loss and good health. The optimal amounts of vitamin D, calcium, and omega-3 fatty acids in particular will help to boost heart health, bone health, brain health, immunity, and more.

YOU WON'T STOP SMILING. I'm willing to bet that your mood has never been better. You are waking ready to face the day—even during those dismal winter months. You're feeling this happy for a reason—and it goes well beyond those skinny jeans that you finally slipped into with ease. Again, the vitamin D and the omega-3 fatty acids work together to boost mood, especially during the long, dark winter months.

YOU FEEL FANTASTIC. Other diets might have left you feeling tired, moody, and listless. Not this one. Again, the D helps to reduce muscle and bone soreness, so you should be feeling more energetic and in the mood to exercise.

THE PLAN WORKS WITH YOUR LIFE—NOT AGAINST IT. Perhaps most important, the 7-Day Slim Down is versatile. You can adapt the plan as needed to suit your lifestyle. You can take it out to eat. You can follow it at dinner parties. And you can mix things up in the name of culinary excitement. From work lunches to a romantic dinner to a Caribbean vacation, you'll be able to take the 7-Day Slim Down with you anywhere so you can stay slim for life.

Rather than sticking to a narrow and rigid set of menu options and eating rules, living the 7-Day Slim Down means that you'll be able to make your own decisions about what and where to eat, where to vacation, what to do on your birthday, and how to celebrate the holidays. Rather than following a set of menus and recipes that I designed for you, you will create your own menus and recipes. Rather than using restaurant suggestions that we came up with for you, you will choose your own eating-out options. In short, you will transition from sitting in the passenger seat on the diet to sitting in the driver's seat as you navigate the rest of your slim and beautiful life.

Three Steps to Become a Lifer

SO NOW YOU have the motivation to become a lifer. Let's talk about how you make that a reality. It's all really very simple. Just keep doing what you are doing. Follow these three steps for a lifetime of success.

STEP #1
KEEP EATING THE SAME MEALS AND THE SAME PORTIONS.

The menus in Chapters 9 through 12 are all calibrated to nourish you with 1,400 to 1,500 calories a day. This number of calories, combined with all of the fat melters in the various dishes should get you all the way to your goal weight. Once you reach your goal, do not change your eating. For 95 percent of you, now is not the time to increase your portions, add another snack, or otherwise increase the amount of food you are eating. That's a recipe for weight gain. There are two exceptions to this basic rule of thumb.

EXCEPTION #1: You're not yet at your goal weight. You'd like to lose more weight, but you've hit a plateau and you can't get past it. Plateaus are frustrating, but they are also often temporary. Most plateaus are actually an illusion caused by slow weight loss. For instance, if you are losing one-quarter pound of fat a week, it will seem as if you are not losing any weight at all. Then, after 4 or so weeks, you'll get on the scale and see that you've dropped a pound. Stay the course for a few weeks and see what happens. You might just start losing again. But If that doesn't work, I recommend you do one of the following:

▶ Decrease your daily calories by omitting one or both daily snacks.
▶ Increase your metabolism by drinking 6 cups of green tea a day.
▶ Start a fitness plan or increase your exercise.

EXCEPTION #2: You've reached your goal but you are still losing. What a good problem to have! In this case, you will want to add a little food back in. It's possible that you are very tall, have a faster than normal metabolism, or are getting a lot more exercise than the average woman. In any case, double up on one or both of your snacks and see what happens.

STEP #2

BECOME A LIFER IN THE KITCHEN.

There are going to be times when you just don't want to follow the menus in this book. During those times you might want to cook your own recipes or design your own meals. That's perfectly fine. I encourage you to make this plan a part of your lifestyle. A big part of success is having the freedom to put your own personal stamp on your eating plan. Use the advice in "Three Steps to Becoming a Lifer in the Kitchen" (page 282) and "The Plate of a Lifer" (page 283) to do just that.

STEP #3

USE YOUR LIFELINES.

There are a few tips and tricks that make weight maintenance a whole lot easier. You'll discover all of them on pages 286 and 287.

Three Steps to Become a Lifer in the Kitchen

IN CHAPTERS 9 THROUGH 13, you found dozens of menus, recipes, and snack suggestions. You can use these options for life. I've made sure to include plenty so you will never feel bored. You can continue to follow these menus and recipes for as long as you'd like.

That said, you will at some point want to adapt your own favorites. When creating your own slimming meals at home, follow these steps.

STEP #1

GIVE YOUR RECIPE A CALORIE SHRINK.

This step is optional, but highly recommended. When you give your recipes a calorie shrink, you are creating the opportunity to consume a bigger portion. With summer dishes, this might not be as important because your appetite during the summer probably isn't as demanding. It's much more important with winter dishes. Swap out full-fat dairy for nonfat or fat-free. Do the same with meat, opting for extra-lean cuts and varieties. For instance, extra-lean ground turkey is a much better option than regular ground beef. As a compromise, consider mixing a lower-fat option with a higher-fat option. For instance, mix lean ground beef with extra-lean ground turkey. Finally, extend higher-calorie ingredients (especially meat) with lower-calorie ones. Experiment by adding chopped veggies or even tofu to various meat dishes. One exception: It's better to consume whole eggs because the D, antioxidants, and omega-3s are all housed in the yolk.

STEP #2

SWAP IN SOME D.

Here are a few ways to pump up the D with various high D foods.

▸ Milk: Add fat-free milk to dishes that call for water. For instance, use it to make a broth-based soup creamy.

▸ D-fortified tofu: Tofu will take on the taste and texture of any dish, making it an extremely versatile way to add more D and drop the number of calories in nearly any recipe. You can mix it into every-thing from lasagna to casseroles to burgers. You can even use silken tofu in smoothies and soups.

▸ Mushrooms: Mushrooms serve as a great topping, filling, and extender. Add them to soups. Use them in sauces. Grind them up to create fillings for burgers, crab cakes, and more.

▸ Egg: Perhaps you can mash up hard-cooked ones and mix them into a cold salad. Or you might mix cooked scrambled egg into soup or a rice casserole.

▸ D-fortified yogurt: Use it in place of sour cream. Add it to smoothies. Use it to give soups a creamy consistency.

STEP #3

CALCULATE THE RIGHT PORTION.

You want your portion to total no more than 400 calories for any given meal. To figure out the correct portions, sign up for a calorie analysis site such as nutritiondata.com. Type your ingredients into the online calculator to get a caloric value for the total meal, then calculate the correct portion from there.

The Plate of a Lifer

Whether you are creating breakfast, lunch, or dinner, use the follow-ing chart on page 284 to ensure that you end up with a D-rich meal. Each meal you consume should include three items: a protein, a wild card (starch *or* dairy *or* nuts *or* healthy fat), and produce. In every meal, at least one of these should be a high-D option. Give yourself bonus points if you create a meal with two high-D options; give yourself a gold star if you manage to include three.

1 PROTEIN + 1 WILDCARD + 1 PRODUCE = SUCCESS

OPTIONS THAT ARE HIGH IN D ARE IN BOLD.

Choose one or more high in D.

PROTEIN

(120–200 cals)

FISH

- **4–5 ounces salmon (sockeye)**
- 4–5 ounces halibut
- 4–5 ounces catfish
- **4–5 ounces tuna (bluefin)**

- **4 ounces steelhead trout (canned)**
- 6 ounces cod (Atlantic)

SHELLFISH

- **6–8 raw Eastern oysters or 3 Pacific oysters**
- ½ pound medium shrimp

MEAT

- 4–5 ounces skinless chicken or turkey breast
- 4–5 ounces lean beef

MISCELLANEOUS

- 6 ounces tofu
- **2 eggs**

WILD CARD

(100–150 cals)

GRAINS

- ½ cup cooked barley
- **2 slices D-fortified bread (1-oz slices)**
- 1 English muffin
- 2 soft flour whole wheat tortillas (6") or 1 soft flour whole wheat tortillas (8")
- ½ cup cooked millet
- ½ cup cooked brown rice
- ¾ cup whole wheat cooked pasta
- 2 mini whole wheat pitas or 1 large whole wheat pita
- **½ cup oatmeal or D-fortified hot cereal (uncooked) or 1 cup D-fortified cold cereal**

ROOT VEGETABLES

- ½ medium potato, baked
- 1 cup diced potatoes
- ¾ cup sweet potato
- 1 medium corn on the cob or ¾ cup kernels

BEANS AND LEGUMES

- ½ cup cooked beans
- ½ cup cooked lentils
- 1 cup peas (sweet, sugar snap)
- ⅔ cup edamame (shelled)

NUTS AND SEEDS

- 1–2 Tbsp nuts or seeds

DAIRY

- 1 oz low-fat cheese
- 2 Tbsp low-fat cream cheese
- **1 cup fat-free milk**
- ¾ cup fat-free or ½ cup reduced-fat ricotta cheese
- ¾ cup 1% or fat-free cottage cheese or ½ cup 2% cottage cheese

HEALTHY FATS

- ½ sliced avocado
- 5 olives, halved
- 1 Tbsp olive oil

PRODUCE

(80-100 cals)

FRUIT

- 1 whole fruit (plum, nectarine, peach, pear, apple)
- 2 or 3 figs
- 1 cup mango
- 2 cups cantaloupe
- 1½ cups honeydew melon
- 2 cups watermelon
- ¼ cup dried fruit
- 1 large banana
- 2 cups mixed berries

RAW VEGETABLES
(UNLIMITED UNLESS OTHERWISE NOTED)

- 1 whole artichoke
- Asparagus
- Bean sprouts
- Bok choy
- Broccoli
- Brussels sprouts
- Cabbage
- Carrots (1 cup)
- Cauliflower
- Celery
- Collard greens
- Cucumbers
- Eggplant
- Green or red peppers
- Iceberg (head) lettuce
- Kale
- Mesclun greens
- **Mushrooms**
- Mustard greens
- Okra
- Onions (½ cup chopped)
- Romaine lettuce
- Spinach
- Tomatoes
- Turnip greens
- Watercress
- Wax beans
- Winter squash (1 cup, 40 calories)
- Zucchini

Your Lifelines for Lasting Success

LIKE THE PHONE-A-FRIEND option on game shows, the following lifestyle strategies will help you find the right answer and stay the course. The longer you maintain your success, the easier maintenance becomes.

DO: IF YOU HAVEN'T ALREADY STARTED A FITNESS PLAN, START ONE NOW. Exercise helps you maintain your success by keeping you in a healthy state of mind. Numerous studies show that people who exercise tend to eat fewer fattening foods and make healthier food choices overall. A study by the National Weight Control Registry found that nearly all of 784 study participants who had lost at least 30 pounds, and had maintained that loss for 1 year or longer, used diet and exercise not only to lose the weight, but also to maintain the weight loss.

DO: STAY VIGILANT. People who weigh themselves are more likely to maintain their weight loss. Getting on the scale regularly—I recommend once a week—gives you important feedback. Another way to measure yourself is just to keep a close eye on how your clothes fit. Are your jeans a bit tight? Maybe you need to cut back. Cocktail dress feels almost a size too big? Make sure you're eating enough, so you avoid a rebound binge.

DO: READ AS MUCH ABOUT HEALTH AND NUTRITION AS YOU CAN. Think of it as bibliotherapy. Subscribe to health magazines (like *Women's Health*) and even read other nutrition books. In addition to helpful advice, your reading will help keep you in a healthy frame of mind.

DO: HANG WITH THE RIGHT FRIENDS WHO SUPPORT YOU. Various studies show that our friends' habits can rub off on us. If you spend time with friends who are overweight, or just tend to eat and gab, it can derail your success. This certainly doesn't mean that you should ignore all of your girlfriends who love food! But be mindful of the time you spend together. Instead of always meeting over dinner or drinks, suggest a walk in the park.

DO: SEEK SUPPORT ONLINE. A University of Vermont study found that dieters who had online weight-loss buddies were better able to maintain their weight loss than dieters who didn't.

DO: COME UP WITH A NEW GOAL. You've lost weight. You've done one of the hardest things any human can do. You are capable of anything and everything. Why stop now? What else can you improve in your life? The more you improve your life, your relationships, your career, and other aspects of personal happiness, the more likely you will remain on the plan. Positive emotions such as joy and contentment have been associated with weight maintenance. The better your life, the better you'll feel, and the more likely you will be to keep off the weight. So pick a new challenge. Put a date on the calendar. Sign up for a 5-K. Plan a great vacation that involves a physical activity like snorkeling or skiing. Find what motivates you and go after it.

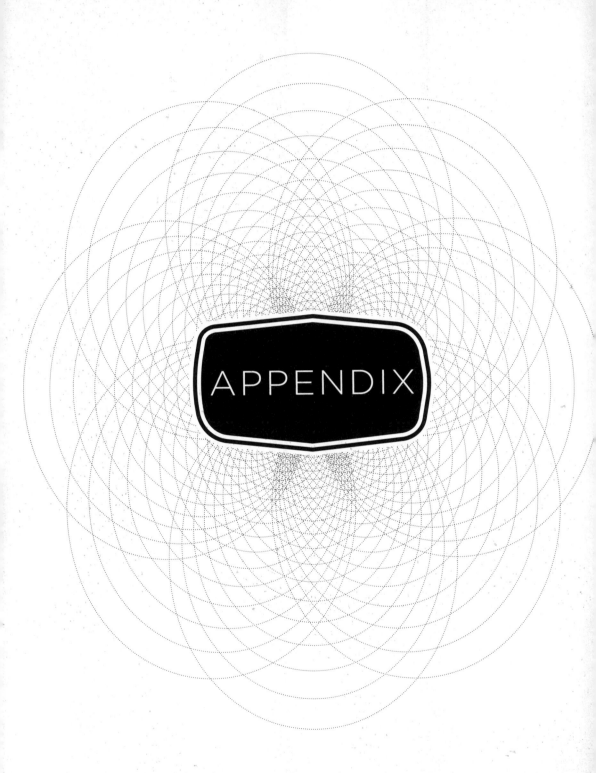

APPENDIX

The Resource List

Many dieters tell me that much of their struggle to lose weight has little to do with cravings, hunger, or even motivation, and everything to do with getting organized. They tell me that they never quite followed their diets correctly because they never got around to finding the right foods, for instance.

I don't want that to stand between you and success. It's my hope that you will find everything you need in this chapter to organize your life and your kitchen for weight loss.

In the following pages you will find many different lists. Most of them are lists of recommended brands of foods. I am not affiliated with any of these brands. I'm only including them here to ease some of the burden of weight loss for you. Rather than tell you to go to the grocery store and read label after label until you find foods that are fortified with D, I've done the sleuthing for you.

Keep in mind that new products hit grocery store shelves every day. The following lists are not exhaustive. If you find a D-fortified food that is not included on a list in this appendix, that doesn't automatically mean it doesn't work with the diet. No, what it probably means is this: The food appeared on the market after my writing deadline for this book had passed.

How to Read Labels for Vitamin D

When reading labels to find foods that work with this plan, you generally want to look for three different numbers:

1) THE NUMBER OF CALORIES PER SERVING

2) THE AMOUNT OF FAT

3) THE PERCENTAGE OF D

None of this is as straightforward, however, as it might initially sound.

Nutrition Facts

Serving Size: 1 Container (113 g)
Servings Per Pack: 4

Amount Per Serving

Calories: 50	Calories from fat: 0

	% Daily Value
Total Fat 0g	0%
Saturated Fat 0g	0%
Trans Fat 0g	0%
Cholesterol less than 5mg	1%
Sodium 55mg	2%
Potassium 150mg	4%
Total Carbohydrate 13g	4%
Dietary Fiber 5g	20%
Sugars 4g	
Protein 3g	6%

Vitamin A	10%	**Vitamin D**	15%
Calcium	10%	**Phosphorus**	8%

Not a significant source of vitamin C and iron
*Percent Daily Values are based on a 2,000 calorie diet.

For instance, let's take a look at the label for Yoplait Fiber One yogurt, which does work with the plan and is a great snack option for you. Here's how to read the label.

LOOK AT THE NUMBER OF CALORIES. Here, you'll see that the yogurt contains 50 calories. Then make sure to look at the number of servings. On this particular product, there is only one serving in the container, so the yogurt offers 50 calories per package. You could eat *two* of these and have them count as just *one* of your daily snacks. Note that, for many products, there are more than one serving per container. In that case, multiply the number of servings by the number of calories to find out how many calories are in a package. For instance, a product that says it has 2.5 servings and 50 calories would contain 125 calories per package.

LOOK AT THE FAT CONTENT. Try to choose nonfat and fat-free versions of all of the dairy products you consume.

LOOK AT THE D CONTENT. You'll find this toward the bottom of the food label, where all of those % signs are. If you do not see D listed at all, that means there is either no D or only a negligible amount of D in the product. If you see D listed, you'll need to do a little math to figure out how much D the product contains. Food labels are somewhat confusing when it comes to vitamin D because they are still based on the old, outdated recommendation from the Institute of Medicine for 400 IU of D. Now the Institute of Medicine recommends 600 IU of D, but the Daily Value listed on food labels is still listed as 400 IU. Therefore, when you see a product that claims to have 30 percent of the DV for D, that means it contains 30 percent of 400 IU, or 120 IU per serving. On the label shown on page 291, it says the product has 15% of the DV for D. To calculate how many IU of D are in the container, multiply the DV (400) by the percentage listed on the label (15%, or 0.15). In this case, the answer is 60 IU.

Top D Foods

From most to least, here's how much D you'll find in a 200-calorie serving of the following foods.

FOOD	IU OF D	FOOD	IU OF D
Cod liver oil	2,217	Corn Flakes	156
Herring, Atlantic	2,061	Kellogg's All-Bran Bran Buds	106
Catfish	1,053	Hot chocolate, homemade, with D-fortified milk	104
Oysters	941		
Salmon, sockeye, canned	920	Kellogg's All-Bran Complete Wheat Flakes	87
Salmon, pink, canned	898	Kellogg's Corn Flakes	84
Steelhead trout	760	Post Bran Flakes	83
Halibut	645	Kellogg's Complete Bran Flakes	83
Sardines	516	General Mills Whole Grain Total	80
Mackerel	351	General Mills Rice Chex	77
Soy milk, fortified, Silk	338	General Mills Almond Crunch with Raisins	77
Shrimp	287		
OJ, fortified	259	Post Grape-Nuts Flakes	76
Milk, fortified	248	New England clam chowder, made with 2% milk	72
Tuna, light, canned	238		
Caviar	184	Banana pudding, made with 2% milk	69
Cod	160	Clams	11

Top D Fish Picks

Fish generally serves as your most concentrated source of D. From highest to lowest, the following fish are all good picks.

1. Salmon, wild
2. Oysters
3. Herring
4. Catfish, channel
5. Halibut
6. Sardines
7. Mackerel
8. Shrimp
9. Tuna, light, canned in water
10. Caviar, black and red
11. Cod

Top Cereal Picks

The following cereals are all high in D, low in sugar, and rich in other important weight-loss nutrients like fiber.

- Cream of Wheat Healthy Grain Instant, original
- Kellogg's All Bran with Extra Fiber
- Kellogg's All-Bran Original
- Malt-O-Meal High Fiber Bran Flakes

- Kellogg's All-Bran Buds
- Kellogg's All-Bran Complete Wheat Flakes
- Post Bran Flakes
- General Mills Whole Grain Total

- Healthy Choice Almond Crunch with Raisins
- Fiber One
- Post Raisin Bran
- Total Wheat Flakes

Top D–Fortified Food Picks

The following list is not comprehensive. It's my hope that more and more D-fortified products have appeared on the market since I constructed this list. Use this list as a guide and for inspiration, but not as a stopping point. If you find a D-fortified product that isn't on this list, by all means, go ahead and use it.

Recommended Brands	Serving Size	Calories per serving	%DV per 2,000 calorie diet	IU per serving
MILK SUBSTITUTES				
Almond Breeze	1 cup	60	25	100
Silk almond milk	1 cup	60	25	100
Silk vanilla soy milk	1 cup	100	30	120
Silk Plus Omega-3 DHA soymilk	1 cup	110	30	120
Organic Valley soy milk	1 cup	110	30	120
WestSoy plain soy milk plus	1 cup	90	25	100
WestSoy rice beverage	1 cup	110	25	100
Tempt hemp milk	1 cup	70–170	25	100

Recommended Brands	Serving Size	Calories per serving	%DV per 2,000 calorie diet	IU per serving
MILK: CHOOSE FAT-FREE WHENEVER POSSIBLE				
Horizon Organic milk (skim)	8 oz	90	25	100
Horizon Organic milk (whole)	8 oz	150	25	100
Farmland Dairies Skim Plus	1 cup	110	25	100
Organic Valley Skim Milk	1 cup	90	25	100
Lactaid	1 cup	90	25	100
Land O'Lakes skim milk	1 cup	90	25	100
Stonyfield Farm Organic Fat-Free milk	1 cup	90	25	100
Carnation Fat-Free	2 Tbsp	25	6	24
Parmalat	1 cup	130	25	100
YOGURT: CHOOSE NONFAT VARIETIES WHENEVER POSSIBLE				
Yoplait Original	6 oz	170	50	200
Dannon Light & Fit	6 oz	80	20	80
Yoplait Fiber One yogurt	4 oz	50	15	60
Stonyfield Farm fat-free plain yogurt	6 oz	80	20	80
Yoplait Light Thick & Creamy	1 container	100	20	80
Yoplait Light	1 container	110	20	80
Breyers Light	6 oz	80	20	80
Stonyfield Farm Fat-Free Activia	4 oz	90	15	60
Yoplait Yo-Plus	4 oz	110	10	40
CHEESE: CHOOSE 1% OR LOW-FAT WHENEVER POSSIBLE				
Kraft Singles	1 slice	45	10	40
BREAD: CHOOSE WHOLE GRAIN WHENEVER POSSIBLE				
Sara Lee Soft & Smooth 100% Whole Wheat Bakery Bread	2 slices	150	15	60
Sara Lee Soft & Smooth made with whole grain white bakery bread	2 slices	150	15	60
Stroehmann whole grain white bread	2 slices	130	10	40
Stroehmann whole wheat bread	2 slices	120	10	40
TOFU				
Vitasoy USA Nasoya Lite Firm Tofu	¼ package	40	30	120
ORANGE JUICE				
Florida's Natural Orange Juice plus calcium with added vitamin D	8 oz	110	25	100
Simply Orange with calcium and vitamin D	8 oz	110	25	100

(continued)

Top D-Fortified Food Picks (cont.)

Recommended Brands	Serving Size	Calories per serving	%DV per 2,000 calorie diet	IU per serving
ORANGE JUICE (CONT.)				
Minute Maid Home Squeezed Style Orange Juice, calcium + vitamin D	8 oz	110	25	100
Tropicana calcium + vitamin D	8 oz	110	25	100
EGGS				
Eggland's Best eggs	1 large	70	20	80
MARGARINE				
Smart Balance Buttery Spread Original	1 Tbsp	80	50	200
Smart Balance Whipped Low-Sodium Buttery Spread	1 Tbsp	60	50	200
Country Crock original spread	1 Tbsp	70	15	60
MUSHROOMS				
Dole Portobello Mushrooms	3 oz	20	100	400
Monterey Mushrooms sliced mushrooms: look for vitamin D claim on select varieties	3 oz	20	100	400
Eden Foods Shiitake Mushrooms, dried	6 slices	35	25	100
COMMERCIAL SMOOTHIES AND BREAKFAST SHAKES				
Pair with a piece of fruit, egg, or cheese stick for a light meal on the run.				
Bolthouse Farms Protein Plus Parfait Smoothie	8 oz	180	2	8
Carnation Breakfast Essentials drink	1 packet	130	25	100
Edy's Slow Churned Shakes	10 oz	210	25	100
BARS				
Pair with a piece of fruit, egg, or cheese stick for a light meal on the run.				
LUNA chocolate peppermint stick	1 bar	180	15	60
LUNA protein, cookie dough	1 bar	170	15	60
Slim Fast chocolate peanut caramel bar	1 bar	200	20	80
Special K protein bar, double chocolate	1 bar	170	4	16
MISCELLANEOUS				
Swiss Miss Great Start Cocoa (add as a snack)	1 envelope	110	20	80
VitaTops Apple Crumb muffin	1	100	50	200
Vitamin Water Stur-D	8 oz	40	10	40

Suggested Restaurant Options

It's difficult to nail down restaurant options in a book because even the chain restaurants change their menus quite regularly and many more do not list vitamin D content as part of their nutritional analysis. As a result, for many of the following meal suggestions, I had to guess the D content based on the ingredients used in the dish.

Some of the following suggestions may not necessarily be high in D, but they are calorie controlled nonetheless. If you do not eat out very often, it's okay to have a low-D option at a restaurant as long as you don't go over your calorie budget. Some of the following meals are higher than your calorie budget. They are in bold. If you opt for any of these suggestions, either hold yourself to just half of a portion or skip one of your snacks that day.

Menu Item	Calories	Estimated D
APPLEBEE'S		
Glazed Shrimp & Spinach	310	1 IU
7-oz House Sirloin topped with sautéed garlic mushrooms	250+130=380	28 IU
5 GUYS		
Little Cheeseburger	**550**	**3 IU**
ARBY'S		
Prime-Cut Chicken Tenders, 3	380	3.5 IU
Roasted turkey breast, 6 oz	220	12 IU
Chocolate milkshake, special	290	123 IU
AU BON PAIN		
Scrambled egg	35	44–80 IU
Tuna and Cheddar on a Farmhouse Roll (half sandwich)	370	68 IU
Tuna Garden Salad	270	68 IU
BENIHANA		
Salmon Roe sashimi	156	250 IU

(continued)

Suggested Restaurant Options (cont.)

Menu Item	Calories	Estimated D
BOB EVANS		
Hardcooked Egg (1 egg)	57	40–80 IU
Scrambled eggs, 2	168	40–80 IU
Fruit & Yogurt Plate	348	2 IU
Salmon Fillet	243	447 IU
Wildfire Salmon Fillet	312	447 IU
Slow-Roasted Chicken Pot Pie	**862**	**9 IU**
BURGER KING		
Cheeseburger	350	3 IU
Chicken Tenders, 6 pc	260	7 IU
CALIFORNIA PIZZA KITCHEN		
Non-Fat Yogurt Smoothies	200-223	2–100 IU
CARL'S JR		
Hand-Breaded Buffalo Chicken Tenders, 3	340	7 IU
Chili Cheeseburger	320	3 IU
CHECKERS		
All-beef hot dog	280	16 IU
CHICK-FIL-A		
Yogurt Parfait	180	2–100 IU
Icedream (small cone)	170	25 IU
CHILI'S		
GG Classic Sirloin	370	8 IU
DENNY'S		
Clam Chowder	266	62 IU
Top Sirloin Steak	220	8 IU
Two-egg breakfast	200	80–160 IU
DUNKIN' DONUTS		
Bacon, Egg & Cheese on English Muffin	370	40–80 IU
Tuna Salad Sandwich on an English Muffin	380	68 IU
FRIENDLY'S		
Homestyle Clam Chowder, cup	270	62 IU
FUDDRUCKERS		
Salmon Filet without bun	**432**	**447 IU**

Menu Item	Calories	Estimated D
HOULIHAN'S		
Tomato Soup with Cheese Fritters	320	62 IU
Grilled 4 oz Atlantic Salmon	332	447 IU
IHOP		
SIMPLE & FIT Spinach, Mushroom & Tomato Omelette with fresh fruit	330	50–90 IU
SIMPLE & FIT Fresh Fruit and Yogurt Bowl	320	2 IU
JACK IN THE BOX		
Hamburger with Cheese (in kid's meal)	330	3 IU
Strawberry Banana Smoothie	290	2 IU
Mango Smoothie	290	2 IU
KFC		
Filet Sandwich without sauce	370	20 IU
OR Chicken Breast	370	3 IU
Crispy strips, 3	380	7 IU
MCDONALD'S		
Cheeseburger	300	3 IU
Filet-O-Fish	380	20 IU
Chicken McNuggets, 6	280	7 IU
Egg McMuffin	300	40–80 IU
Mango Pineapple Smoothie	350	2 IU
Fruit 'n Yogurt Parfait	160	2 IU
NOODLES & COMPANY		
Tomato Basil Bisque, small	280	62 IU
The Med Salad (small) with sautéed shrimp	240	1 IU
OLIVE GARDEN		
Herb-Grilled Salmon	**510**	**447 IU**
P.F. CHANG'S		
Asian Grilled Norwegian Salmon (half a serving)	345	447 IU
PANDA EXPRESS		
Crispy Shrimp, 6	260	2 IU
Golden Treasure Shrimp	390	2 IU
Honey Walnut Shrimp	370	2 IU
PANERA		
Creamy Tomato Soup	310	62 IU
Strawberry Granola Parfait	310	2 IU

(continued)

Suggested Restaurant Options (cont.)

Menu Item	Calories	Estimated D
PANERA (CONT.)		
Half Tuna Salad Sandwich on Honey Wheat	260	68 IU
Egg & Cheese on Ciabatta	390	50–90 IU
Breakfast Power Sandwich on Whole Grain	340	50–90 IU
POPEYE'S		
Butterfly Shrimp, 8	290	2 IU
Popcorn Shrimp	330	4 IU
Louisiana Nuggets, 6	230	7 IU
QUIZNOS		
Tuna Melt Bullet	350	68 IU
Tomato Basil Soup, bowl	160	62 IU
RED LOBSTER		
Manhattan Clam Chowder, bowl	160	62 IU
Broiled Seafood Platter	300	4 IU
Grilled Shrimp Skewers, lunch	360	1 IU
Grilled, broiled, or blackened halibut	280	196 IU
Grilled, broiled, or blackened rainbow trout, lunch	220	645 IU
Grilled, broiled, or blackened salmon, lunch	270	447 IU
Grilled, broiled, or blackened tuna	360	70 IU
Grilled, broiled, or blackened cod	300	20 IU
RUBY TUESDAY		
Petite Jumbo Shrimp Scampi	374	1 IU
Clam Chowder	318	62 IU
Grilled Salmon	350	447 IU
Berry Good Yogurt Parfait	162	2 IU
SIZZLER		
Fried Shrimp, 6	267	2 IU
SONIC		
All-beef regular hot dog	330	16 IU
Jr. Breakfast Burrito	340	40–80 IU
STARBUCKS		
Tuna Salad Bistro Box	380	68 IU
Strawberry and Blueberry Yogurt Parfait	300	2 IU

Menu Item	Calories	Estimated D
SUBWAY		
Tuna Mini Sub with cheese	320	68 IU
Sausage & cheese, English muffin with eggs	290	40–80 IU
Sunrise Subway Melt	230	40–80 IU
6" Cheese Omelet Sandwich	380	50–90 IU
New England Clam Chowder	150	62 IU
Cream of Mushroom soup	160	62 IU
Yogurt Parfait	150	2 IU
TONY ROMA'S		
Seared ahi tuna	365	70 IU
WENDY'S		
Jr. Cheeseburger Deluxe	350	3 IU
WHITE CASTLE		
Cheeseburger	170	3 IU
Sausage, Egg, and Cheese on a bun	320	40–80 IU
ZOUP!		
Chicken Potpie soup	210	9 IU
Tomato Basil soup	150	62 IU
Seafood Chowder	230	62 IU

ENDNOTES

INTRODUCTION

Ginde AA, Liu MC et al. "Demographic differences and trends of vitamin D insufficiency in the US population, 1988-2004." *Archives of Internal Medicine.* (2009 March 23); 169(6): 626–32.

Gilsanz V, Kremer A, et al. "Vitamin D status and its relation to muscle mass and muscle fat in young women." *The Journal of Clinical Endocrinology & Metabolism* (2010 April);95(4): 1595–601.

CHAPTER ONE

Swinburn B, Ravussin E. " Energy balance or fat balance." *American Journal of Clinical Nutrition* (1993); 57 (suppl): 766S–71S.

Cannell JJ, Hollis BW, Sorenson MB, Taft TN, Anderson JJ. "Athletic performance and vitamin D." *Medicine and Science in Sports and Exercise* (May 2001), 41 (5): 1102–10.

CHAPTER TWO

Hess AF. "The Prevention and Cure of Rickets by Sunlight." *American Journal of Public Health* (1922 February);12(2): 104–7.

Beyonddiscovery.org/content /view.txt.asp?a=414

Norman AW. "Minireview: vitamin D receptor: new assignments for an already busy receptor." *Endocrinology.* (2006 December);147(12): 5542–48.

Goodwin PJ, Ennis M, et al. "Prognostic effects of 25-hydroxyvitamin D levels in early breast cancer." *Journal of Clinical Oncology.* (2009 August 10);27(23): 3757–63.

Morimoto S, Yoshikawa K. Psoriasis and vitamin D3. "A review of our experience." *Archives of Dermatology.* (1989 February);125(2): 231–34.

Gilbert-Diamond D, Baylln A, Mora-Plazas C, Arsenault JE, Hughes MD, Willett WC, Villamor E. "Vitamin D deficiency and anthropometric indicators of adiposity in school-age children: a prospective study," *American Journal of Clinical Nutrition.* (December 2010) 92 (6): 1445–51.

Van Rossum CT, Shipley MJ, et al. "Seasonal variation in cause-specific mortality: are there high-risk groups? 25-year follow-up of civil servants from the first Whitehall study." *International Journal of Epidemiology* (2001 October);30(5): 1109–16.

Lee DM, Tajar A, et al. "Association between 25-hydroxyvitamin D levels and cognitive performance in middle-aged and older European men." *Journal of Neurology, Neurosurgery & Psychiatry.* (2009 July); 80(7): 722–29.

Robinson PD, Högler W, et al. "The re-emerging burden of rickets: a decade of experience from Sydney." *Archives of Disease in Childhood* (2006 July); 91(7): 564–68.

Ginde AA, Liu MC et al. "Demographic differences and trends of vitamin D insufficiency in the US population, 1988-2004." *Archives of Internal Medicine.* (2009 March 23); 169(6): 626–32.

Pearce SH, Cheetham TD. "Diagnosis and management of vitamin D deficiency." *British Medical Journal.* (2010 January 11); 340: b5664.

CHAPTER THREE

Jain R, von Hurst PR, et al. "Association of vitamin D receptor gene polymorphisms with insulin resistance and response to vitamin D." *Metabolism.* (2011 August 24).

Nikooyeh B, Neyestani TR, Farvid M, Alavi-Majd H, Houshiarrad A, Kalayi A, Shariatzadeh N, Gharavi A, Heravifard S, Tayebinejad N, Salekzamani S, Zahedirad M. "Daily consumption of vitamin D- or vitamin D + calcium-fortified yogurt drink improved glycemic control in patients with type 2 diabetes: a randomized clinical trial." *American Journal of Clinical Nutrition* (2011 April 93) (4): 764–71.

Kamycheva E, Sundsfjord J, Jorde R. "Serum parathyroid hormone level is associated with body mass index." *European Journal of Endocrinology* (2004 August) 151 (2): 167–72

A. R. Josse, S. A. Atkinson, M. A. Tarnopolsky, S. M. Phillips. "Increased Consumption of Dairy Foods and Protein during Diet- and Exercise-Induced Weight Loss Promotes Fat Mass Loss and Lean Mass Gain in Overweight and Obese Premenopausal Women." *Journal of Nutrition.* (2011); 141 (9): 1626 DOI: 10.3945/jn.111.141028

Mason C, Xiao L, et al. "Effects of weight loss on serum vitamin D in postmenopausal women." *The American Journal of Clinical Nutrition* (2011 July); 94(1): 95–103.

Compston JE, Vedi S, et al. "Vitamin D status and bone histomorphometry in gross obesity." *The American Journal of Clinical Nutrition.* (1981 November);34(11): 2359–63.

Bell NH, Epstein S, et al. "Evidence for alteration of the vitamin D-endocrine system in obese subjects." *The Journal of Clinical Investigation.* (1985 July);76(1): 370–73.

Wortsman J, Matsuoka LY, et al. "Decreased bioavailability of vitamin D in obesity." *The American Journal of Clinical Nutrition.* (2000 September); 72(3): 690–93.

Sibley S. "Plasma Vitamin D: A Predictor of Subsequent Weight Loss Success," presented at The Endocrine Society's 91st Annual Meeting in Washington, D.C. June 2009.

Kamycheva E, Joakimsen RM, et al. "Intakes of calcium and vitamin d predict body mass index in the population of Northern Norway." *The Journal of Nutrition.* (2003 January); 133(1): 102–6.

Krishnaveni GV, Veena SR, Winder NR, Hill JC, Noonan K, Boucher BJ, Karat SC, Fall CH. "Maternal vitamin D status during pregnancy and body composition and cardiovascular risk markers in Indian children: the Mysore Parthenon Study." *American Journal of Clinical Nutrition* (2011 March) 93 (3): 628–35.

Gilbert-Diamon D, Baylin A, Mora-Plazas M, Marin C, Arsenault JE, Hughes MD, Willett WC, Villamor E. "Vitamin D deficiency and anthropometric indicators of adiposity in school-age children: a prospective study." *American Journal of Clinical Nutrition* (2010 December) 92 (6): 1446–51.

Lindgärde F, Ercilla MB, et al. "Body adiposity, insulin, and leptin in subgroups of Peruvian Amerindians." *High Altitude Medicine & Biology.* (2004 Spring); 5(1): 27–31.

Schmitt LH, Harrison GA. "Patterns in the within-population variability of stature and weight." *Annals of Human Biology* (1988 September-October); 15(5): 353–64.

Kamycheva E, Sundsfjord J, Jorde R. "Serum parathyroid hormone level is associated with body mass Index." *European Journal of Endocrinology* (2004 August) 151 (2): 167–72.

Gilsanz V, Kremer A, et al. "Vitamin D status and its relation to muscle mass and muscle fat in young women." *The Journal of Clinical Endocrinology & Metabolism.* (2010 April); 95(4): 1595–601.

Zemel MB, Richards J, Mathis S, Milstead A, Gebhardt L, Silva E. "Dairy augmentation of total and central fat loss in obese subjects." *International Journal of Obesity.* (2005) 1–7.

Heaney RP, Davies KM, et al. "Calcium and weight: clinical studies." *Journal of the American College of Nutrition.* (2002 April); 21(2): 152S–5S.

Major GC, Alarie FP, et al. "Calcium plus vitamin D supplementation and fat mass loss in female very low-calcium consumers: potential link with a calcium-specific appetite control." *The British Journal of Nutrition.* (2009 March); 101(5): 659–63.

Caan B, Neuhouser M, et al. "Calcium plus vitamin D supplementation and the risk of postmenopausal weight gain." *Archives of Internal Medicine.* (2007 May 14); 167(9): 893–902.

Mojtahedi MC, Thorpe MP, et al. The effects of a higher protein intake during energy restriction on changes in body composition and physical function in older women. *The Journals of Gerontology Series A: Biological Sciences and Medical Sciences.* 2011 November;66(11): 1218–25.

Kabir M, Skurnik G, Naour N, Pechtner V, Meugnier E, Rome S, Quignard-Boulangé A, Vidal H, Slama G, Clément K, Guerre-Millo M, Rizkalla SW. "Treatment for 2 mo with n 3 polyunsaturated fatty acids reduces adiposity and some atherogenic factors but does not improve insulin sensitivity in women with type 2 diabetes: a randomized controlled study." *American Journal of Clinical Nutrition.* (2007 December); 86(6): 1670–79.

Rasmussen LG, Larsen TM, Mortensen PK, Due A, Astrup. "Effect on 24-h energy expenditure of a moderate-fat diet in monounsaturated fatty acids compared with that of a low-fat, carbohydrate rich diet: a 6 mo controlled dietary intervention trial." *American Journal of Clinical Nutrition* (2007 April); 85 (4): 1014–22.

Larsen DA, Harmansen K, Stender S, Holst JJ, Tourbro S, Martinussen T, Astrup A. "Comparison of the effects on insulin resistance and glucose tolerance of 6-mo high-monounsaturated-fat, low-fat, and control diets." *American Journal of Clinical Nutrition* (2008 April); 87 (4): 855–62.

Paniagua JA, Gallego de la Sacristana A, Romero I, Vidal-Puig A, Latre JM, Sanchez E, Perez-Martinez P, Lopez-Miranda J, Perez-Jimenez F. "Monounsaturated Fat–Rich Diet Prevents Central Body Fat Distribution and Decreases Postprandial Adiponectin Expression Induced by a Carbohydrate-Rich Diet in Insulin-Resistant Subjects." *Diabetes Care,* (July 2007) 30 (7): 1717–23.

Johnston CS. "Strategies for Healthy Weight Loss: From Vitamin C to the Glycemic Response," *Journal of the American College of Nutrition.* (2005) vol 24 no 3: 158–65.

Wang Y, Jones P. "Dietary conjugated linoleic acid and body composition." *American Journal of Clinical Nutrition.* (2004) 79 (Suppl): 1153S–58S.

Norris LE, Collene AL, Asp ML, Hsu JC, Liu LF, Richardson JR, Li D, Bell D, Osei K, Jackson RD, Belury MA. "Comparison of dietary conjugated linoleic acid with safflower oil on body composition in obese post menopausal women with type 2 diabetes." *American Journal of Clinical Nutrition* (2009 September) 90 (3): 468–76.

Close RN, Schoeller DA, Watras AC, Nora EH. "Conjugated linoleic acid supplementation alters the 6-mo change in fat oxidation during sleep." *American Journal of Clinical Nutrition.* (2007) 86: 797–804.

Gaullier JM, Halse J, Hoivik HO, Hoye K, Syvertsen C, Nurminiemi M, Hassfeld C, Einerhand A, O'Shea M, Gudmundsen O. "Six months supplementation with conjugated linoleic acid induces regional-specific fat mass decreases in overweight and obese." *British Journal of Nutrition.* (2007) 97: 550–60.

Snitker S, Fujishima Y, Shen H, Ott S, Pi-Sunyer X, Furuhata Y, Sato H, Takahashi M. "Effects of novel capsinoid treatment on fatness and energy metabolism in humans: possible pharmacogenetic implications." *American Journal of Clinical Nutrition* (2009) 89: 45–50.

Chen YK, Cheung C, et al. "Effects of Green Tea Polyphenol (-)-Epigallocatechin-3-gallate on Newly Developed High-Fat/Western-Style Diet-Induced Obesity and Metabolic Syndrome in Mice." *Journal of Agricultural and Food Chemistry.*" (2011 October 18).

CHAPTER FOUR

Frost M, Abrahamsen B, Nielsen TL, Hagen C, Andersen M, Brixen K. "Vitamin D status and PTH in young men: a cross-sectional study on associations with bone mineral density, body composition and glucose metabolism." *Clinical Endocrinology.* (2010 November) 73 (5): 573–80.

Taheri S, Lin L, Austin D, Young T, Mignot E. "Short sleep duration is associated with reduced leptin, elevated ghrelin, and increased body mass index." *PLOS Online* (December 2004).

Eliasson A, Kashani M, Turner E, Vernalis M. "Sleep is a critical factor in the maintenance of a healthy weight." presented at the June 2009 SLEEP conference.

Patel SR, Malhortra A, White DP, Gottlieb DJ, Hu F. "Association between reduced sleep and weight gain in women." *American Journal of Epidemiology.* 164 (10): 947–54.

Johnston CS. "Strategies for Healthy Weight Loss: From Vitamin C to the Glycemic Response." *Journal of the American College of Nutrition.* (2005) 24 (3):158–65

Andrade AM, Greene GW, Melanson KJ. "Eating slowly led to decreases in energy intake within meals in healthy women." *Journal of the American Dietetic Association.* (2008 July) 108 (7): 1186–91.

Zijlstra N, de Wijk RA, Mars M, Stafleu A, de Graaf C. "Effect of bite size and oral processing time of a semisolid food on satiation." *American Journal of Clinical Nutrition.* (2009 August) 90 (2): 269–75.

CHAPTER FIVE

Schleithoff SS, Zittermann A, et al. "Vitamin D supplementation improves cytokine profiles in patients with congestive heart failure: a double-blind, randomized, placebo-controlled trial." *The American Journal of Clinical Nutrition.* (2006 April); 83(4): 754–59.

Milaneschi Y, Shardell M, et al. "Serum 25-hydroxyvitamin D and depressive symptoms in older women and men." *The Journal of Clinical Endocrinology and Metabolism.* (2010 July); 95(7): 3225–33.

Gloth FM 3rd, Alam W, et al. "Vitamin D vs broad spectrum phototherapy in the treatment of seasonal affective disorder." *The Journal of Nutrition, Health & Aging.* (1999); 3(1): 5–7.

Lansdowne AT, Provost SC. "Vitamin D3 enhances mood in healthy subjects during winter." *Psychopharmacology.* (1998 February); 135(4): 319–23.

Logan AC. "Omega-3 fatty acids and major depression: a primer for the mental health professional." *Lipids in Health & Disease.* (2004 November 9); 3: 25.

Gloth FM 3rd, Alam W, et al. "Vitamin D vs broad spectrum phototherapy in the treatment of seasonal affective disorder." *The Journal of Nutrition, Health & Aging.* (1999); 3(1): 5–7.

Cannell JJ, Holliss BW, Sorenson MB, Taft TN, Anderson JJ. "Athletic performance and vitamin D." *Medicine and Science in Sports and Exercise.* (May 2009) 41 (5): 1102–10.

Turner MK, Hooten WM, et al. "Prevalence and clinical correlates of vitamin D inadequacy among patients with chronic pain." *Pain Medicine.* (2008 November); 9(8): 979–84.

Goldstone T. Presentation: "Stomach hormone ghrelin increases desire for high-calorie foods." *The Endocrine Society* (2010, June 20).

Havermans RC, Salvy SJ, Jansen A. "Single-trial exercise-induced taste and odor aversion learning in humans."*Appetite.* (2009 August 25).

Burke LE, Sereika SM, Music E, Warziski M, Styn MA, Stone A. "Using instrumental paper diaries to document self-monitoring patterns in weight loss." *Contemporary Cinical Trials.* (2008 March 29) (2): 182–93.

Burke LE, Styn MA, Glanz K, Ewing JJ, Elci OU, Conroy MB, Sereika SM, Acharya SD, Music E, Keating AL, Sevick MA. "SMART trial: a randomized controlled clinical trial of self-monitoring in behavioral weight management-design and baseline findings." *Contemporary Clinical Trials.* (2009 August 7). Wansink B, van Ittersum K, Painter JE. "Ice cream illusions bowls, spoons, and self-served portion sizes." *American Journal of Preventative Medicine.* (2006 September 3) (3): 240–43.

Wansink B, Painter JE, North J. "Bottomless bowls: why visual cues of portion size may influence intake." *Obesity Research.* (2005 January 13) (1): 93–100.

Van Gucht D, Vansteenwegen D, Beckers T, Hermans D, Baeyens F, Van den Bergh O. "Repeated cue exposure effects on subjective and physiological indices of chocolate craving." *Appetite.* (2008 January) 50(1): 19–24.

Hetherington MN, Foster R, Newman T, Anderson AS, Norton G. "Understanding variety: tasting different foods delays satiation." *Physiology and Behavior.* (2006 February 28); 87 (2): 263–71.

Carraca E.V. et al. "Body image change and improved eating self-regulation in a weight management intervention in

s KS. "Increasing
educes risk of
ns in women."
n. (2009 March)

CHAPTER SEVEN

P, et al.
min D
nd fat mass loss
-calcium
ial link with a
ppetite control."
Nutrition. (2009
-63.

. "Helping
themselves."
Nutrition
: 89–96.

CHAPTER EIGHT

et al. "Demo-
s and trends of
ncy in the US
004." Archives
e. (2009 March

al. "Effects
erum vitamin D
women."
f Clinical
); 94(1): 95–103.

CHAPTER FOURTEEN

N, Jakicic JM,
JW, Smith BK .
cal activity
ies for weight
of weight
American
edicine.
ce in Sports
February);

N
79–

Hunter GR, Brock DW et al.
"Exercise training prevents regain
of visceral fat for 1 year following
weight loss." Obesity (Silver
Spring). (2010 April); 18(4):
690–95.

Whybrow S, Hughes DA, Ritz P,
Johnstone AM, Horgan GW, King
N, Blundell JE, Stubbs RJ. "The
effect of an incremental increase in
exercise on appetite, eating
behavior and energy balance in
lean men and women feeding ad
libitum.". British Journal of
Nutrition. (2008 November);
100(5): 1109–15.

King NA, Caudwell PP, Hopkins M,
Stubbs JR, Naslund E, Blundell JE.
"Dual-process action of exercise
on appetite control: increase in
orexigenic drive but improvement
in meal-induced satiety." American
Journal of Clinical Nutrition. (2009
October); 90(4): 921–27.

Levine JA. "Nonexercise activity
thermogenesis—liberating the
life-force." Journal of Internal
Medicine. (2007 September);
262(3): 273–87.

CHAPTER FIFTEEN

Klem ML, Wing RR, et al. "A
descriptive study of individuals
successful at long-term maintenance of substantial weight loss."
American Journal of Clinical
Nutrition. (1997 August); 66(2):
239–46.

Harvey-Berino J, Pintauro S, et al.
"Effect of internet support on the
long-term maintenance of weight
loss." Obesity Research. (2004
February); 12(2): 320–29.

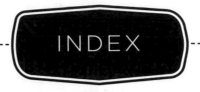

INDEX

Underscored page references indicate sidebars and tables.
Boldface references indicate photographs.

C

Calcium
  blocking iron absorption, 6
  deficiency of, 27
  food sources of, 96, 98, 103, 105
  in 4-Week Slim Down, 111, 160
  functions of, 27
  as mood booster, 81
  provided for prehistoric creatures, 22, 23
  in restaurant meals, 164
  in 7-Day Slim Down, 46, 47, 138
  as slimmer, 10, 53–54, 98, 116, 116
  tracking intake of, 116–17
  vitamin D increasing absorption of, 23, 27, 28, 54, 116
Calorie burning
  from exercise, 251
  from fat cells, 45
  MUFAs improving, 55
  from muscle, 9, 46–47, 57, 256
  from protein vs. fat, 3–4
Calories
  in beverages, 162, 199
  extra, weight gain from, 3
  on food labels, 291, **291**
  in 4-Week Slim Down, 163
  in menus, 58, 112, 280
  reducing, for handling plateaus, 281
  in restaurant foods, 163, 163
  in 7-Day Slim Down, 138
  in Summer Light Menus, 198
  in Winter Warming soups, 191
Calorie shrinking, for recipes, 282
Cancer. See also Skin cancer
  overweight and, 50
  vitamin D and, 28, 29, 33
Cantaloupe
  Lox, Eggs, and Onions with Toast and Cantaloupe, 174
Capsaicin
  as optional slimmer, 57
  in 7-Day Slim Down, 142
Carbohydrates
  allowed in 7-Day Slim Down, 4, 12–13
  muscle burning, 46, 47
Cardio exercise prescription, 255–56
Carrots
  Seared Shrimp with Stir-Fried Vegetables, 240
  Spicy Tuna in a Pita with Carrots, Tomatoes, and Avocado, 180
  Wild Mushroom and Beef Stew with Wild Rice and Carrots, 193

Catfish
  Catfish Fingers with Spicy Mayonnaise, 233
  Catfish Fingers with Spicy Mayonnaise and Sweet Potato, 194
Cauliflower
  Orange Poached Salmon with Star Anise, Spinach, and Roasted Cauliflower, 194
Cayenne, for speeding metabolism, 190
Cereals
  Almond Butter Toast with Yogurt and Granola Crunch, 173
  Banana-Nut Hot Cereal, 172
  Cereal with Strawberries and Almonds, 144, 150, 156, 172
  vitamin D–rich, 294
  whole grain breakfast, 106
CFS, 83
Cheating, on diets
  exercise preventing, 247
  in 4-Week Slim Down, 166
  inevitability of, 76
  90/10 principle about, 16
  slowing weight loss, 162, 189
Cheese. See also Mozzarella cheese; Parmesan cheese
  vitamin D in, 295
Chicken
  Chicken Cacciatore, 218
  Chicken Cacciatore with Sautéed Escarole, 177
  Chicken in a Skillet with Couscous, 177
  Chicken Scallopini with Garlic Mushroom Sauce, 230
  Chicken Scallopini with Garlic Mushroom Sauce and Artichoke, 193
Chocolate
  Chocolate Mocha Smoothie, 211
Cholesterol, blood, omega-3 fatty acids improving, 96
Chowder
  Salmon and Corn Chowder, 239
  Salmon Corn Chowder and Salad, 203
Chronic fatigue syndrome (CFS), 83
Cinnamon, 72, 99
CLA, as slimmer, 56
Clothing, for winter warmth, 191
Cod liver oil, as cure for rickets, 26
Coffee
  Chocolate Mocha Smoothie, 211
  Hazelnut Latte, 211
Coleslaw
  Portobello Sandwich with Coleslaw, 183
Comfort foods, 11, 85–86

N

O

Weight lifting. *See* Strength training
Weight loss. *See also* Diets
  expected, from 7-Day Slim Down, 10, 58,
    111, 138
  maintaining, xiii, 103, 111, 248, 286–87
  misleading information about, 2, 3
  motivation for (*See* Motivation)
  for releasing vitamin D stored in fat, 131
  of 7-Day Slim Down participants, 19, 39, 59
  sleep for, 71
  slowed by cheating, 162, 189
  slowing metabolism, 11, 112
  soup for, 191
  stress reduction for, 71, 72
  summer, xi
  support for, 86–87, 286–87
  vitamin C for, 105–6
Weight loss plateaus, 11, 280–81
Wellbutrin, for Seasonal Affective Disorder,
  82
Whey protein, in dairy products, 98
Whole grain bread, as fat-melting food, 103–4
Whole grain breakfast cereal, as fat-melting
  food, 106
Whole grain crackers
  Beef Barley Soup and Whole Grain
    Crackers, 193
Wild rice
  Wild Mushroom and Beef Stew with Wild
    Rice and Carrots, 193
Willpower, xii, 77–78. *See also* Motivation
Wine, 3, 12, 14, 141, 162
Winter
  depression in, xi, xiii, 79–82, 79, 80, 190
  fatigue in, 83–84
  reduced sunlight in, 78, 83, 188, 253
  vitamin D deficiency during, xii, 48–49
  weight gain during, x–xi, xii, 2, 48–49, 52
Winter Warming Menus, 18, 80, 86, 111, 120, 121
  features of, 188–89
  how to follow, 189
  menus, 161, 193–95
  recipes
    Beef Barley Soup, 228
    Beef Barley Soup and Whole Grain
      Crackers, 193
    Broiled Mackerel, 236
    Broiled Mackerel in Lemon Mint Sauce
      with String Beans Almondine, 195
    Catfish Fingers with Spicy Mayonnaise,
      233

Catfish Fingers with Spicy Mayonnaise
  and Sweet Potato, 194
Chicken Scallopini with Garlic
  Mushroom Sauce, 230
Chicken Scallopini with Garlic
  Mushroom Sauce and Artichoke,
  193
Halibut with Asparagus and Shiitake
  Mushrooms, 234
Halibut with Asparagus and Shiitake
  Mushrooms and Roasted Potatoes,
  194
Miso Soup with Tofu and Shrimp, 235
Miso Soup with Tofu and Shrimp and
  Edamame, 195
Orange Poached Salmon with Star
  Anise, Spinach, and Roasted
  Cauliflower, 194
Orange Poached Salmon with Star
  Anise and Spinach, 232
Sesame-Crusted Salmon, 231
Sesame Crusted Salmon with Green
  Beans and Tomato Salad, 194
Stuffed Portobello Mushrooms, 237
Stuffed Portobello Mushrooms with
  Roasted Butternut Squash, 195
Wild Mushroom and Beef Stew, 229
Wild Mushroom and Beef Stew with
  Wild Rice and Carrots, 193
soup in, 191, 192
supercharging, 190–91
"Wonder vitamins," 5–6, 49
Wrinkles, sunscreen preventing, 36

Y

Yoga, before bed, 271–72
Yogurt
  Almond Butter Toast with Yogurt and
    Granola Crunch, 173
  Berry Yogurt with Scrambled Eggs, 148,
    154, 173
  cereal mixed with, 106
  as sauce, 99
  vitamin D in, 99, 283, 295
  Waffles, Yogurt and Sparkling OJ, 173

Z

Zinc absorption, soy hindering, 6